Contents

Introduction

Because an increasing number of young children today do not have the opportunity to take part in regular play, physical activity or exercise, enjoyable, vigorous, well taught physical education lessons are more important than ever. Equally important is a sense of staff unity regarding the 'Why?', the 'What?', and the 'How?' of physical education to deliver a whole school, successful programme with continuity and high standards from year to year. The main reasons for teaching physical education, include:

Physical development. First and foremost, the main reason for teaching physical education has always been to inspire vigorous, enjoyable, challenging and wholehearted physical activity that develops normal healthy growth and satisfactory development of each pupil's strength, suppleness and stamina. The skills taught also aim to develop skilful, confident, well-controlled and safe movement. It is hoped that the varied skills will give pleasure and satisfaction, catering for many interests and aptitudes, and will eventually enable pupils to take part in healthy, worthwhile and sociable activities long after they have left school. These skills, learned and enjoyed at school, are remembered by the body for a very long time.

Personal, social and emotional development, compensating for the near total disappearance of play in the out-of-school lives of many of our pupils. It is reported that millions of children spend most of their free time – up to five hours every day – watching a TV or a computer screen. It has also been claimed that parents, who refuse to let their children go out to play, are producing a 'battery-farmed' generation who will never become resilient and will be unable to deal with risk.

This lack of play means no exercise, no fresh air, no physical development, no social development though interaction with others, no adventure in challenging situations and no emotional development. It has been said 'an individual's regard for, and attitude to, his or her physical self, especially at primary school age, is important to the development of self-image and the value given to self.' Physical education lessons are extremely visual, providing many opportunities for demonstrating success, creativity, versatility and enthusiastic performances which should be recognised by the teacher, praised and commented upon, and shared with others who should be encouraged to be warm in their praise and comments. Such successes can enhance a pupil's feelings of pride and self-confidence.

The play-like nature of physical education lessons is obvious. In games, running, jumping and landing, throwing and catching, batting, skipping, trying to score points or goals; in gymnastic activities, running, jumping and landing, rolling, climbing, swinging on ropes, balancing, circling on bars; and in dance, skipping, running and jumping, travelling with a partner, a group or a circle in performing a dance, are all playful actions in which pupils find fun and satisfaction from performing well, and social development from being in the company of others.

When teaching physical education lessons now, teachers need to remember that the lessons may be providing the only active play that some of the pupils will experience that week. The lessons must be vigorous, enjoyable, and give an impression of children at play.

Contributing to pupils' health now, and long after they have left school. The health of our children and eventually the health of our nation, has been a cause for concern for university researchers and health experts for decades. A 1997 headline described British children as 'The Flab Generation'. It was estimated in 2000, that in a class of thirty children, two will go on to have a heart attack, three will develop diabetes, and thirteen will become obese, all as result of a sedentary lifestyle and a diet dominated by chips, biscuits, sweets and sugary drinks. A 2002 report revealed that a third of 10 year olds did not even walk continuously for ten minutes a week.

The above statistics and figures have become far worse since those early ignored warnings. The NHS treated 85,000 patients for clinical obesity in 2007 and a 2008 report from the NHS Information Centre claims that 'a third of children between the ages of 2 and 15 are now obese or overweight'. England has the fastest growing weight problem in Europe. The link between obesity and diabetes is well known and 100,000 UK patients are diagnosed with type 2 diabetes every year, fuelled by the nation's obesity problem. Douglas Smallwood, Chief Executive of the charity Diabetes UK says 'Diabetes is a serious condition which can lead to devastating complications such as blindness, amputation, heart and kidney disease.' Almost one hundred diabetics a week have a limb amputated because of complications with their disease.

An extra twelve kilograms in weight boosts the risk of cancer by 50%. Coronary heart disease causes 105,000 deaths a year and 2.6 million people are thought to be living with the symptoms of heart disease. Scientists have warned that unfit, lazy children are six times more likely to develop early signs of heart disease than those who are active and take exercise. For the first time, experts have established that activity levels in children as young as seven can have a serious effect on their future health. Professor Paul Gately, of Leeds Metropolitan University says 'Inactive children at a relatively young age are already storing up health risks for the future.' Health specialists, concerned for the health of our nation, are now repeatedly emphasising the importance of regular exercise as the best way to reduce the risks of suffering life-threatening illnesses in later life.

The National Obesity Forum has called for urgent action to tackle the obesity problem which, they calculate, causes 30,000 deaths each year and emphasises that the time to act is in childhood before irreversible damage has been done, and while lifelong habits can be learned. British Heart Foundation research found that taking 30 minutes of moderate exercise most days reduces the risk of an early death by more than a quarter. Diabetes UK warns that obesity is making a diabetes epidemic inevitable. Physical activity and a sensible diet are the best ways to reduce the risk of developing diabetes. The World Cancer Research Fund 2007 Report, produced by scientists and medical experts from around the world, tells us that most cancers are preventable by choosing a healthy diet, being physically active and maintaining a healthy weight. They recommend being physically active for at least 30 minutes every day, to keep the heart healthy and to reduce the risk of cancer.

Realistically, it is only in schools in physical education lessons, that we can encourage and help children to succeed in a wide range of physical skills and inspire, motivate and facilitate a joy in physical activity that will combat the health problems mentioned above. Physical education makes a unique contribution to an all-round, balanced education, but it also makes a special contribution to a life-prolonging, healthy lifestyle. For today's primary school children regular, excellent, vigorous and enjoyable physical education lessons are probably the best health products they will ever receive.

Teaching Physical Education

The teacher of physical education, almost uniquely, works alone and unaided, and is involved in whole class teaching with no help from the mass of teaching aids that help to keep pupils purposefully and often independently engaged in their classrooms. Even if he or she is talking to an individual, a pair or a small group, the teacher in a physical education lesson still needs to be aware of the whole class and how it is responding to the set task.

The teacher is the source and inspiration for everything that happens in the lessons. He or she needs to be well prepared to make the lesson complete, enjoyable, stimulating and challenging; enthusiastic to create an equally enthusiastic response; warm and encouraging to help pupils feel pleased and good about themselves; and intensely interested in inspiring vigorous physical activity in pupils, many of whom, away from school, may have inactive and sedentary lifestyles.

The lesson plan is the teacher's essential guide and reminder of the current lesson's content. Failure to plan and record lessons results in the same or similar things being done, month after month. Parts of the lesson gradually disappear, and an unprepared teacher can finish up doing no teaching in a lesson where everything is vague or has been done before. Pupils at apparatus in such an unprepared lesson answer 'Nothing' when asked 'What has your group been asked to do at this apparatus?'

July's lesson will only be at a more advanced stage that the previous September's if all the lessons in between have been recorded and referred to, to make each succeeding lesson move on and introduce new, interesting and exciting challenges. The lesson usually runs for four or five weeks (one lesson per week) to give the class enough time to practise, improve, develop, learn, remember and enjoy all the skills involved.

'Dead spots' and queue avoidance. The 'scenes of busy activity' which every physical education lesson should be requires an understanding by all pupils that they should be 'found working, not waiting'. This means that they need to be trained to respond immediately, behave well, keep on practising until stopped, and avoid standing immobile in queues.

The teacher needs to avoid talking the class out of their lesson through over-long explanations, demonstrations and pupil reflections following demonstrations. Lessons that lose a lot of time result in unsatisfactory, hurried apparatus work, frustratingly short time for playing games, and half-created dances with no time to share them proudly, with the class.

Demonstrations and observations by pupils and teacher are essential teaching aids because we remember what we see – good quality work; safe, correct ways to perform; the exact meanings of physical education terminology; and good examples of variety and interesting contrasts. All can watch one, two or a small group. Half of the class can watch the other half. Each can watch a partner. These occasional demonstrations, with comments by the observing pupils, often bring out good points not noticed by the teacher; train pupils to understand the elements of 'movement'; and let teachers ask 'how can it be improved?' Making friendly, encouraging, helpful points to classmates is good for class morale and for extending the class repertoire in physical education. ('Occasional' means once or twice at most in one lesson because of the time taken to do this.)

Further class practice should always follow a demonstration so that everyone can try to include some of the good features praised and commented on.

Shared choice or **indirect teaching** takes place when the teacher decides the nature of the activity and challenges the class to decide on the actions. Limits set are determined by the experience of the pupils. From the simple 'Can you travel on the apparatus, using your hands and feet?' with its slight limitations, we can progress on to 'Can you travel on the apparatus, using hands and feet, and include a still balance, a direction change, and taking all the weight on your hands at some point?'

Shared choice teaching produces a wide variety of results to add to the class repertoire. Being creative is extremely satisfying and most primary school pupils enjoy and are capable of making individual responses.

Direct teaching takes place when the teacher tells the class what to do, including, for example: any of the traditional gymnastic skills; the way to hold, throw and catch a ball; or how to do a folk dance step. Correct, safe ways to move; support yourself; grip, lift and carry apparatus; and throw implements, are all directly taught.

If the class is restless, not responding, or doing poor work, a directed activity can restore interest and discipline and provide ideas and a valuable starting point from which to develop. Pupils who are less interested, less inventive or less gifted physically, will benefit from direct teaching, particularly if the teacher can suggest an alternative, simpler but equally acceptable idea. 'If you do not like rolling forwards, try rolling sideways instead. Start, curled up on your back, with your hands clasped under your knees. This keeps your head out of the way.' The occasional stimulus of a direct request is the kind of challenge many pupils enjoy, and they respond enthusiastically. 'Can you and your partner bat the small ball up and down between you, six times?'

Motivational teaching. Children say that the things that motivate them to take part in physical activities are fun and skill development. They want to enjoy, learn and succeed. The more philosophical among them might also add that feelings of happiness are associated with having something to look forward to; to enjoy; and then to remember with pleasure (and often with pride). This anticipation, realisation and retrospect-inspiring potential of excellent physical education lessons and activities, makes it the favourite subject for many primary school pupils.

Safe Practice and Accident Prevention

In physical education lessons, where a main aim is to contribute to normal, healthy growth and physical development, we must do everything possible to avoid accidents.

Good supervision by the teacher is key to safe practice. He or she must be there with the class at all times, and teaching from positions from which the majority of the class can be seen. This usually means circulating on the outside looking in, with no-one behind his or her back. Good teaching develops skilful, well-controlled, safe movement with pupils wanting to avoid others to ensure that they have space to practise and perform well and not be impeded in any way. The outward expression of this caring attitude we are trying to create is the sensible, unselfish sharing of hall floor space, apparatus and playground, and self-control in avoiding others.

Badly behaved classes who do not respond immediately, or start or stop as requested; who rush around selfishly and noisily disturbing others; who are never quiet in their tongues or body movements; and who do not try to move well, are destructive of any prospects for high standards or lesson enjoyment by the majority and the teacher. A safe environment requires a well-behaved, quiet, attentive and responsive class. Good behaviour must be continually pursued until it becomes the normal, expected way to work in every lesson. There is nothing to talk about, apart from those occasions when comments are requested after a demonstration, or when partners are quietly discussing their response to a challenge.

The hall should be at a good working temperature with windows and doors opened or closed to cope with changing seasons and central heating variations. Potentially dangerous chairs, tables, trolleys, piano or television should be removed or pushed against a wall or into a corner. Floor sockets for receiving securing pins for ropes and climbing frames should be regularly cleared of cleaning substances which harden and block the small sockets.

In playground games lessons, pupils must be trained to remain inside the lines of the grids or netball courts and to avoid running, chasing or dodging into fences, walls, sheds, seats, hutted classrooms, or steps into buildings. In any 'tag' games, pupils must be told 'Touch the person you have caught very gently, never pushing them or causing them to fall or stumble.'

Before the lesson, the teacher checks for sensible, safe clothing with no watches, rings or jewellery whose impact against another child can cause serious scarring or injury; no long trousers that catch heels; no long sleeves that catch thumbs, impeding safe gripping; and no long, un-bunched hair that impedes vision. Indoors, barefoot work is recommended because it is quiet, provides a safe, strong grip on apparatus, enhances the appearance of the work, and enables the little-used muscles of feet and ankles to develop as they grip, balance, support, propel and receive the body weight.

In teaching gymnastic activities, the following safety considerations are important:

○ In floor and apparatus work, pupils need to be taught the correct, safe, 'squashy' landing after a jump so that they land safely on the balls of the feet, with ankles, knees and hips 'giving' without jarring.

○ When inverted, with all the weight on their hands, pupils need to be taught to keep fingers pointing forward, arms straight and strong, and head looking forward, not back under arms. Looking back under the arms makes everything appear to be upside down.

○ On climbing frames, pupils must be told 'Fingers grip over the bar, thumbs grip under the bar, always, for a safe, strong grip.'

Headings When Considering Standards in Physical Education

Physical Education lessons are so visual that most of the following headings can be considered by an interested observer.

○ **Vigorous physical activity**, involving all pupils for most of the lesson, is the most important feature of an excellent lesson.

○ **Responsive pupils, behaving well and obviously enjoying lessons**; working hard to learn and improve skills; and exuding enthusiasm and concentration, are an uplifting feature of high standards.

○ **Enthusiastic teaching, using praise and encouragement warmly**, stimulates pupils to even greater levels of endeavour. Praise is specific, referring to what is pleasing, to inform the pupil being praised and to let others hear and learn. 'Well done, Susan. Your balances are still, firm and beautifully stretched.'

○ **Skills, appropriate to the age group, are taught and developed**. There is an impression of skilful, quiet, confident, well-controlled, successful performing with economy of effort. Pupils show understanding by their ability to remember and repeat their movements.

○ **Pupils' behaviour towards one another is excellent**. Undressing and dressing quickly to extend lesson time; safe, unselfish sharing of space and apparatus; working quietly to avoid lessons being stopped because of noise; observing demonstrations with interest and then making helpful, friendly comments; and co-operating well as partners and members of groups and teams, all indicate desirable standards of behaviour.

○ **Varied teaching styles include**:

    a indirect or shared choice teaching

    b direct teaching

    c good and varied use of demonstrations, observations, comments.

○ **Satisfactory time allocation** provides regular, weekly lessons in dance, games and gymnastic activities – a broad programme which also includes athletic activities and swimming for Juniors.

○ **Lesson plans** are in evidence, as a reminder of all parts of the current lesson, and as a reminder of what has been taught, so that the work can be progressed, month by month, throughout the year.

○ **Sensibly dressed pupils** wear shorts, a T shirt or blouse, and plimsolls. Indoors, barefoot work is recommended. As an example, the teacher should at least change into appropriate footwear.

○ **Continuity and progression from year to year** are evident in the way that older pupils work harder for longer at increasingly difficult activities, demonstrating skill and versatility.

○ **An awareness of safe practice and accident prevention** is evident in the way that pupils share the limited space. The correct way to lift, carry and use apparatus, land, move, roll, support and use the body generally, are regularly mentioned.

A Suggested Way to Start a First Lesson With a New Class

Unless taught otherwise, pupils travel round the hall or the playground in an anti-clockwise circle, all following the person in front of them. If one pupil slows down or stops suddenly, the next can bump into that person, possible knocking him or her over, causing an angry upset and a disturbance.

By travelling and confining themselves within this circle, a class fails to use all the possible room or playground space, depriving themselves of enough space to travel freely in different directions, and to join several actions together, on the spot or travelling about. Also, with everyone travelling round in a circle, sometimes side by side, pairs of less well-behaved pupils can be so close together that their poor behaviour, expressed in talking, not listening, slow responses, and noisy, poor performances, completely upsets the teacher's aim to give the class an enjoyable, lively, quiet, thoughtful and co-operative start to the lesson and the year's programme.

By continually making the whole class listen for the signal 'Stop!', we force them to pay attention, listen, and respond quickly.

Suggested pre-start to the lesson

1 Please show me your very best walking...go! Visit every part of the room, the sides, the ends, corners, as well as the middle. Swing your arms strongly and step out smartly.

2 When I call 'Stop!', show me how quickly you can stop and stand perfectly still. Keep walking smartly and visiting all parts of the room. Stop! Stand still!

3 If you are standing too near a piece of apparatus, like Liam by the piano, or too near someone else, like Thomas and Emily, please take one step into a big space all by yourself. Go!

4 When you start walking this time, travel along straight lines, never following anyone. If you find yourself behind someone, change direction and continue along a new straight line, following no-one. Ready? Go!

5 Come on. March briskly and smartly and pretend you are leaving footprints in every part of the room. When I call 'Stop!' you will stop immediately and then take a step into your own space if you are near apparatus or another person. Stop!

6 In our next practice, listen for my 'Stop!' and show me that no-one is standing behind another person, looking towards that person's back, following them. Go!

7 Stop! Stand still, after moving onto your own space if necessary. Now show your very best running, with the emphasis on lifting your heels, knees and hands to keep your running soft, silent and strong – and, of course, travelling along straight lines, never following anyone.

8 Stop! Be still! This half of the class stand with feet apart, arms folded, to watch this other half doing their very best running. Look out for and tell me later about anyone whose running you liked and be able to tell me what you liked about it. The running half...ready...go! Do not pick anyone who is following someone, or anyone who is not lifting heels, knees or arms strongly. Please watch carefully.

9 Stop! Watchers, whose running did you like. Yes, Daniel?

10 I (Daniel) liked Kate's running because she used her eyes well, looking for spaces, and she seemed to float along beautifully and easily, with heels, knees and hands being lifted high.

11 Thank you very much, Daniel, for that excellent answer. Now let's look at Kate to see and learn from the good things mentioned by Daniel. Please run again, Kate.

12 (Repeat with the other half working and the other half observing and commenting.)

Potential Cross-Curricular Outcomes of Physical Education Lessons for Juniors

Language Many teachers recognise the valuable contribution that physical education lessons can make to language development and a clearer understanding of the meanings of words. Hearing, reading and writing are the usual relationships between pupils and words. In physical education lessons, pupils do, experience and feel the action words concerned. Clear demonstrations by the teacher or a pupil also lead to a greater understanding of the exact meanings of action words.

In Year 3, Games Lesson 2, for example, there are: run, side-step, avoid, count, touch, walk, throw, catch, bounce, receive, pass, move, invent, develop, advance, change, practise, revise, show and skip. Jog, sprint, bowl, dodge, mark, chase, aim, reach, land, dribble and receive are also frequently used in games lessons.

In a typical gymnastic activities lesson, pupils will also experience, understand and feel the meanings of the many prepositions used, for example, in Year 4, Lesson 3: over, through, on, astride, along, upward, off, across, up to, from, near, away. Beside, beneath, towards, around, are also used frequently in gymnastics lessons.

Adverbs describe the quality or degree of effort in an action as in Year 5, Dance Lesson 9: vigorously, firmly, slowly, lively, lightly, loosely, stiffly, clearly and loudly. Quickly, gently, strongly, smoothly, suddenly, silently, smartly, carefully, splendidly and explosively, are also used frequently in dance lessons.

Writing Still within language, pupils can be challenged to complete 'The part(s) of the gymnastics lesson where I felt (choose one of) for example, excited, pleased, surprised, tired, proud, anxious, hot, breathless, strong, stretched, sociable, unsure, relaxed, was/were...' They can be asked to try to explain why they were experiencing the feelings that they listed.

A mountaineer once said 'When I climb, I can feel life effervescing within me.' A pupil who has just completed a rope climb for the first time; or done a beautifully controlled handstand, then lowered into a forward roll; or completed their own created dance or gymnastic sequence with complete control from start to finish, with attractive use of space and effort; or outwitted a close marking opponent, before going on to score, will be experiencing intense excitement, pride and pleasure, deserving of the opportunity to try to produce an eloquent expression about what might have been an unforgettable event.

Art They can be asked 'Can you draw the gymnastic action or actions that gave you the most pleasure or excitement in today's lesson? Under your heading, can you explain in a few words why you were pleased or excited?'

Physical Education can also contribute to pupils':

○ **spiritual development** through helping them gain a sense of achievement and develop positive attitudes towards themselves

○ **moral development** through helping pupils gain a sense of fair play based on rules and the conventions of activities; and develop positive sporting behaviour, knowing how to conduct themselves in sporting competition

○ **social development** through helping pupils develop social skills in activities involving co-operation and collaboration, responsibility, personal commitment, loyalty and teamwork, and considering the social importance of physical activity, sport and dance.

Gymnastic Activities

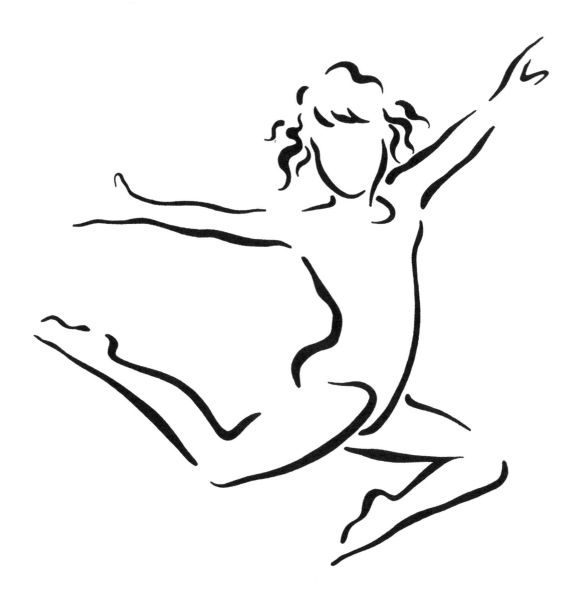

Introduction to Gymnastic Activities

Gymnastic Activities is the indoor lesson that includes varied floorwork on a clear floor, unimpeded by apparatus, followed by varied apparatus work which should take up just over half of the lesson time. Ideally, the portable apparatus will have been positioned around the sides and ends of the room, near to where it will be used, before lessons start in the morning or afternoon. This allows each of the seven or eight mixed infant groups, or the five or six mixed junior groups of pupils to lift, carry and position their apparatus in a very short time, because no set will need to be moved more than 3–5 metres. The lesson is traditionally of 30 minutes duration.

The following pages aim, first of all, to produce a sense of staff-room unity regarding the nature of good practice and high standards in teaching Gymnastic Activities lessons. Without this sense of unity among the teachers concerned, there is no continuity of aims, expectations or programme, and there will be a less than satisfactory level of achievement. Secondly, the following pages provide a full scheme of work for Gymnastic Activities. There is a lesson plan and accompanying pages of detailed explanatory notes for every month, designed to help teachers and schools with ideas for lessons that are progressive.

Why We Teach Gymnastic Activities

Ideally, the expressions of intent known as 'Aims' should represent the combined views of all the staff.

Aim 1 To inspire vigorous physical activity to promote normal healthy growth and physical development. Physical Education is most valuable when pupils' participation is enthusiastic, vigorous and wholehearted. All subsequent aims for a good programme depend on achieving this first aim.

Aim 2 To teach physical skills to develop skilful, well-controlled, versatile movement. We want pupils to enjoy moving well, safely and confidently. Physical Education makes a unique contribution to a child's physical development because the activities are experienced at first hand by doing them.

Aim 3 To help pupils become good learners as well as good movers. Knowledge, understanding and learning are achieved through a combination of doing, feeling and experiencing physical activity. Pupils are challenged to think for themselves, making decisions about their actions.

Aim 4 To develop pupils' self-confidence and self-esteem by appreciating the importance of physical achievement; by helping them to achieve; and by recognising and sharing such achievement with others.

Aim 5 To develop desirable social qualities, helping pupils get on well with one another by bringing them together in mutual endeavours. Friendly, co-operative, close relationships are an ever-present feature of Physical Education lessons.

Aim 6 To provide opportunities for exciting, almost adventurous actions (particularly climbing, swinging, balancing, jumping and landing) and vigorous exercise – seldom experienced away from school. We want our pupils to use these lessons as outlets for their energy and we want them to believe that exercise is good for you and your heart, and makes you feel and look better. We aim to encourage participation in a healthy lifestyle, long after pupils have left school.

The Gymnastic Activities Lesson Plan for Juniors – 30–35 minutes

One answer to the question 'What do we teach in a gymnastic activities lesson?' might be – 'All the natural actions and ways of moving of which the body is capable and which, if practised wholeheartedly and safely, ensure normal, healthy growth and physical development.'

It has been said that 'What you don't use, you lose.' Most pupils hardly ever use their natural capacity for vigorous running; jumping and landing from a height; rolling in a different direction; balancing on a variety of body parts; upending to take their weight on their hands; gripping, climbing and swinging on a rope; hanging, swinging or circling on a bar; or whole body bending, stretching, arching and twisting.

These natural movements and actions should be present in every gymnastic activities lesson, ensuring that pupils do not lose the ability to do them and have their physical development diminished.

A teacher's determination to inspire the class to use and not lose their natural physicality can be strengthened by observing how many children are collected in cars at the school gates. They are then transported home to their after school, house-bound, sedentary home lives.

Floorwork (12–15 minutes) starts the lesson and includes:

○ Activities for the legs, exploring and developing the many actions possible when travelling on feet, and ways to jump and land.

○ Activities for the body, including the many ways to bend, stretch, rock, roll, arch, twist, curl, turn, and the ways in which body parts receive, support and transfer the body weight in travelling and balancing.

○ Activities for the arms and shoulders, the least used parts of our body. We strengthen them by using them to hold all or part of the body weight on the spot or moving. This strength is needed in gripping, climbing, hanging, swinging and circling, and in levering on to and across apparatus, supported by the hands alone.

Apparatus Work (16–18 minutes) is the climax of the lesson, making varied, unique and challenging physical demands on pupils whose whole body – legs, arms and shoulders, back and abdominal muscles – has to work hard because of the more difficult tasks:

○ travelling on hands and feet, over, under, across and around obstacles, as well as vertically, often supported only on hands

○ jumping and landing from greater heights

○ rolling on to, along, from and across apparatus

○ balancing on high or narrow surfaces

○ upending to take all body weight on hands on apparatus above floor level

○ gripping, swinging, climbing and circling on ropes and bars.

Final Floor Activity (2 minutes) after the apparatus has been returned to its starting places around the sides, ends and corners of the hall, brings the whole class together again in a simple activity based on the lesson's main emphasis or theme. After the bustle of apparatus removal – the swishing of ropes along trackways, the creaking of climbing frames being wheeled away, the bumping of benches, planks, boxes and trestles – there is a quiet, calm, thoughtful and focused ending.

Three Ways to Teach Apparatus Work

1   **(Easiest Method) Pupils use all the apparatus freely, as they respond to tasks that relate to the lesson theme**. Several challenges provide non-stop apparatus work for infants and juniors. Pupils are stationary only when watching a demonstration, having a teaching point emphasised, or when being given the next task. This method is normally used with infant classes, because they are able to visit and use all pieces of apparatus, including their favourites – ropes and climbing frames.

    'Show me a still balance and beautifully stretched body shape on each piece of apparatus.' (Body shape awareness and balance)

    'Show me how you can approach each piece of apparatus going forward and leave going sideways.' (Space awareness – directions)

    'Leader, show your partner one touch only on each piece of apparatus, then off to the next piece.' (Partner work)

2   **Groups stay and work at one set of apparatus**. Repetition helps pupils improve and remember a series of linked actions. The task is the same for all groups, based on the lesson theme.

    'Make your hands important in arriving on, and your feet important in leaving the apparatus.' (Body parts awareness)

    'Can you include swings on to and off apparatus; a swing into a roll; and a swing to take all the weight on your hands?' (Swinging)

    'Travel from opposite sides, up to, on, along and from the apparatus, to finish in your partner's starting place.' (Partner work)

    Groups rotate to the next apparatus after about five minutes and will work at three sets in a lesson, rotating clockwise one lesson, and anti-clockwise the next, to meet all apparatus every two lessons.

3   **Each group practises a different, specific skill on each piece of apparatus - balancing, rolling, climbing, for example**. This method of teaching is more difficult than the other two because it needs more technical knowledge, and because the teacher is giving five or six sets of instructions instead of one. As it is a direct challenge to 'skills hungry' pupils, it is very popular.

    Benches 'At upturned benches, slowly balance and walk forward. Look straight ahead. Feel for the bench before you step on it.'

    Ropes 'Grip strongly with hands together and feet crossed. Can you take one hand off, while swinging, to prove a good foot grip?'

    Low cross box 'A face vault is like a high bunny jump to cross the box, as you twist over, facing the box top all the way.'

    Climbing frames 'Travel by moving hands only, then feet only.'

    Mats 'Roll sideways with body curled small and then with body long and stretched' (log roll).

    Groups rotate to the next piece of apparatus after about five minutes, rotating clockwise one lesson, and anti-clockwise the next lesson, meeting all apparatus every two lessons.

Organising Groups For Junior School Apparatus Work

Groups of five or six pupils are appropriate for junior school apparatus work, and pupils are placed in their mixed groups in the first lesson in September. Pupils are told 'These are your groups and starting places for apparatus work.' For the four or five sessions' development of a lesson, the same groups go to the same starting places, becoming more expert in lifting, carrying and placing their apparatus in that position.

From their regular starting positions, groups rotate clockwise, probably with time to work at three different sets of apparatus. At the end of the apparatus work, groups return to their own apparatus to move it back to the sides and ends of the room from which it was originally carried. The floor is now clear for the incoming class. In the next lesson, the groups will move anti-clockwise to work at the other three sets of apparatus.

This recommended system for ensuring that apparatus can be lifted, carried and placed in position quickly and easily, needs the co-operation of all the teachers. Before the lessons start in the morning or afternoon, the portable apparatus is placed around the sides and ends of the hall adjacent to where it will be used. Each group will only have to carry it 2–3 metres. A well-trained class can have the apparatus in place in 30 seconds. After all lessons are finished each day, as much of the apparatus as possible should remain in the hall, in corners, against or on the platform, or at the sides and ends of the room. Mats can be stored vertically behind frames, benches and boxes.

Positioning of Apparatus During Lessons

The teacher needs to provide varied actions and different physical demands as pupils progress from apparatus to apparatus to meet a challenging, interesting series of tasks which include:

a climbing and swinging on ropes

b rolling on mats, from benches, along low box

c balancing on inverted benches, planks, along low box

d running and jumping on to mats, across, along and from benches

e climbing on climbing frames

f taking weight on hands on mats, benches, planks, low boxes

g jumping and landing from a height from a bench or box

h circling or hanging from metal pole between trestles

i lying and pulling along a bench or down an inclined plank.

A safe environment is ensured by providing:

a mats where pupils are expected to land from a height

b mats that are well away from walls, windows, doors or other obstacles such as a piano, trolleys or chairs, and well away from the landing areas of adjacent apparatus

c height and width of apparatus that are appropriate for the age of the class – not too narrow to balance on, and not too high to jump from.

Mats are used to cushion a landing from a height and to roll on. We do not need mats under ropes or around climbing frames because we do not ask pupils to jump down from a height. If mats are placed around climbing frames, pupils often behave in a foolhardy way, enticed into dangerous jumping.

Fixed and portable apparatus

In the lesson plans that follow, the equipment continually being referred to and shown in the apparatus layouts includes the following items:

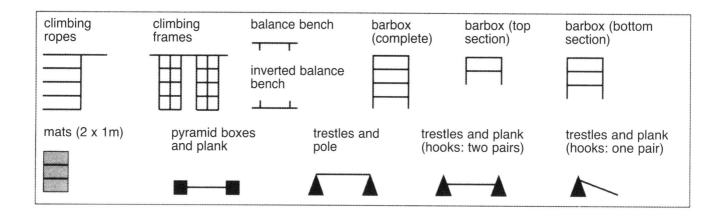

Minimum number recommended:

- 12 mats 2 × 1 m
- 3 balance benches
- 1 barbox that can be divided into two smaller boxes by lifting off the top section; the remaining lower section should have a platform top fitted
- 1 pair pyramid boxes and one plank
- 1 pair of 0.9 m, 1 m, and 1.4 m trestles
- 1 metal pole to join pairs of trestles
- 2 planks with two pairs of hooks
- 2 planks with one pair of hooks

A Pattern for Teaching and Improving A Gymnastic Activities Action

Using 'Travelling' as an example

1 **Quickly into action**. With few words, clearly explain the task and challenge the class to start. For example 'Can you plan to travel, using your feet, sometimes going forwards, and sometimes in another direction?'

2 **While class is working**. Emphasise the main points, one at a time. There is no need to stop a well-behaved class who are working quietly every time you need to make a teaching point. 'Find quiet spaces in all parts of the room – the sides, ends, corners, as well as the middle.' 'Work so quietly that I can't hear you.' 'Travel on straight lines, never curving round, following someone.' 'Look over your shoulder if going backwards.'

3 **Identify and praise good work while class is working**. The teacher needs to circulate round the outside of the room, looking in to see as much of the work as possible. 'Well done, Thomas. I liked your skipping forwards and bouncing sideways.' 'Nathalie, your hopscotch is a great idea.' 'Sarah, your slow, careful running backwards with high knees lifting, is a neat, safe way to travel.'

4 **Demonstrations accompanied by teacher comment are the quickest way to increase the class repertoire**. It saves time if the demonstrators have been told what aspect of movement they are about to be asked to demonstrate. 'We will be looking at your beautifully stretched body in your jumps, and the soft, quiet way you let your knees and ankles give when you land.' 'Stop and watch Daniel's lively, quiet bouncing with feet parting and closing, going sideways. And look at Charlotte's galloping backwards with a strong arm swing.'
   Beware of stopping the class too often to use a demonstration. Make these stoppages brief, between 12 and 15 seconds.

5 **Further practice should follow a demonstration with reminders of the good things seen**. Pupils enjoy copying something they never thought of trying – particularly when it has been warmly praised and approved of. 'Thank you for those excellent demonstrations. Practise again, and try to improve your travelling by using something of what you have just seen. Use your whole body strongly, but quietly. Your feet can travel together or apart, or one after the other.'

6 **Demonstrations (by an individual, a small group or half of the class) with follow-up comments by the pupils are used to let pupils reflect on and evaluate their own and others' performances**. Such comments and judgements guide the next stage of planning for improvement. 'Watch this group of four working and tell me which travelling actions you like best, and say which directions you saw being used.' This is followed by a brief look at the pupils mentioned.

7 **Demonstrators and those making comments are thanked and more class practice lets them try some of the good things seen**. Beware of using demonstrations with follow-up comments more than once or twice in the lesson because they are time-consuming.

Progressing Gymnastic Activities over the 4 or 5 weeks of the Lesson's Development

Using 'Stepping' as an example of an activity to be developed

Lessons 1 and 2

a Concentrate on the **'What?'**, the actions, their correct form, and how the body parts concerned are working.

'Can you step quietly and neatly, visiting all parts of the room? Travel on straight lines, never following anyone.'

'Which parts of the foot can support you? Tip toes, insides or outsides? Long or short steps or a mixture?'

'Can you vary the idea of stepping, not always passing your feet?' (Chasse, crossover, toes down and swing.)

b Insist on good, clear body shapes to make everything look better and be more demanding.

'Step out nice and tall as you travel. Can you show me your clear arms, legs and body shape? Are you long and stretched or is there a body shape change somewhere?'

Lessons 2 and 3

Concentrate on the **'Where?'** of the movement, adding variety and quality by good use of own and whole floor space, directions and levels.

'Can you sometimes step on the spot, (particularly when you are in a crowded area) and sometimes use the whole room space – sides, corners, ends as well as middle.'

'Stepping actions sideways and backwards can be interesting – sliding, stepping-closing (chasse) or cross-stepping over, as well as feet passing normally. The leading leg can swing in many directions.'

Lessons 3 and 4

Consider the **'How?'** of the movements and the way that changes of speed and effort (force) might make the work look more controlled and neat, as well as giving them greater variety, contrast and interest.

'Within your stepping, can you include a change of speed? It might be slow, slow; quick, quick, 3, 4; slow, slow. Flat, flat; tip toes, tip toes, 3, 4; flat, flat.. This is interesting if a change of direction accompanies the speed change. Side, slow, slow; forward, quick, quick, 3, 4; side, slow, slow.' 'Can you make parts of your travelling small, soft, quiet, and make parts bigger, firmer, stronger?' (On the spot, keep it soft, 1, 2, 3, 4; on the move, big strong strides, 1, 2, 3, 4.)

Lessons 4 or Lessons 4 and 5

Ask for **sequences** that draw together all the practising, learning, adapting and remembering that have taken place during the previous lessons and aim for almost non-stop action, working harder for longer with enthusiasm, understanding and concentration.

'In your 3 or 4 part sequence, can you include: varied stepping actions, interesting use of space, and a change of speed or force somewhere?'

The Use of Themes in Teaching Gymnastic Activities

Week after week, month after month, the teacher and class come into the school hall and see the same apparatus, apparently offering the same limited set of activities every time. In dance, we continually move on to learning and performing new dances and building a huge repertoire. In games, the new seasons bring their different sports and the varied games implements provide an interesting and exciting range – including new games created by the teacher and pupils.

Gymnastic activities lessons are made different through applying a new idea, emphasis or theme each month. We do not simply 'do' the basic action. We do it, focusing on a particular aspect of movement, to improve in understanding and versatility, as well as in competence. A theme is a particular aspect of movement chosen by the teacher as a focal point around which to build a series of lessons.

At the very beginning of the series of four or five lessons during which an individual lesson is repeated, it is recommended that the pupils are 'put in the picture' regarding their lesson's main aims or emphases. In cases where they are going to be assessed on the outcome of the lesson, it is essential to explain to them what new skills, knowledge and understanding they will be expected to demonstrate. Identifying the lesson theme or main emphasis to the class is also a way for the teacher to put him or herself 'in the picture' about the main objectives of the lesson and to focus on them.

Start of year themes with a new class, will have an emphasis on good behaviour; sensible, safe sharing of floor and apparatus space; immediate responses to commands and challenges set by the teacher; establishing a tradition of wholehearted, vigorous effort and a co-operative attitude towards one's classmates; and co-operating with others to lift, carry and place apparatus quietly, sensibly and safely.

A suggested set of six progressive themes for a month to month programme

1   **Body parts awareness** for better controlled, safer, more correct activity. 'Show me varied ways to travel, using one foot, both feet, or one foot after the other.'

2   **Body shape awareness** for improved poise, better posture and firmer body tension. 'Can you run and jump up high with feet together and long, straight legs?'

3   **Space awareness** for improved variety, quality and interest, and safer practising. 'Can you travel all round the room, using feet only, sometimes going forwards, and sometimes sideways?'

4   **Effort awareness** for more interesting contrasts, better quality and stronger work. 'As you travel in a variety of ways can you include actions that are small, light and gentle, and actions that are large, lively and strong?'

5   **Sequences** for longer, harder, versatile work, stamping it with own personality. 'Make up a sequence you can remember, of three or four joined-up actions and changing body shapes on different body parts.' (Standing, kneeling, lying, sitting, upended on shoulders, arched on back or front.)

6   **Partner work** for new, enjoyable, sociable, more demanding experiences not possible on one's own, and to extend movement understanding because you need to recognise partner's actions. 'Stand, facing each other. Can you, with a little bend of knees as a start signal, bounce at the same speed? Can you do opposites, with one going up as the other comes down?'

A Progressive Series of Themes for a Gymnastic Activities Programme

An example from parts of lessons based on 'ways to travel'

Floorwork

Apparatus Work

Theme 1. Body parts awareness – for neater, better controlled, safer, more correct activity.

Floorwork

a Show me varied ways to travel, using one foot, both feet, or one foot after the other. As you travel about, slowly, using hands and feet, can you make different parts of your body go first?

Apparatus Work

a Plan to visit many pieces of apparatus. 'Feel' the different ways your hands and feet can:
 1 support you (for example, as you hang, swing, crawl, circle, roll, slide, skip, jump, balance.)
 2 go from apparatus to apparatus, putting hands on the apparatus, and show me a bunny jump with straight arms and well bent legs.

Theme 2. Body shape awareness – for improved poise, better posture and firmer body tension.

Floorwork

a Can you run and jump up high with feet together and long, straight legs?
b Can you run and jump up high to show me a wide shape like a star?

Apparatus Work

a Run quietly round the room, not touching any apparatus. When I call 'Stop!', show me a clear body shape on the nearest apparatus.
b Run round again and when I stop you next time, show me a different, firm body shape.

Theme 3. Space awareness – for improved variety, quality and interest, and safer practising.

Floorwork

a Can you travel all round the room, using feet only, sometimes forwards, and sometimes going sideways? Which are best for going forwards? Which are best for going sideways?

Apparatus Work

a Can you arrive on and leave the apparatus at different places and in different ways?
b Take weight on hands, with straight arms and bent legs. Bring feet down slowly in a new floor space.

Theme 4. Effort awareness – for more interesting contrasts, better quality, and stronger work.

Floorwork

As you travel in a variety of ways, can you include actions that are small, light and gentle, and actions that are large, lively and strong?

Apparatus Work

Travel freely. Show me strong, firm balances on apparatus that contrast with easier travelling actions in between. Can you do a vigorous upward jump, off, then a soft 'giving' landing.

Theme 5. Sequences – for longer, harder, versatile work, stamping it with own personality.

Floorwork

Work in a small floor space and show me two or more ways to travel on feet or feet and hands. Can you give each action a name? Show me a still start and finish.

Apparatus Work

Start in a still, nicely balanced position on the floor. Travel on to a piece of apparatus and show me a neat, still balance position.

Theme 6. Partner work – for new, more exciting experiences not possible on your own.

Floorwork

Follow your leader's varied travelling.

Apparatus Work

Follow on to and along each piece of apparatus.

National Curriculum Requirements for Gymnastic Activities – Key Stage 2: The Main Features

'The government believes that two hours of physical activity a week, including the National Curriculum for Physical Education and extra-curricular activities, should be an aspiration for all schools. This applies to all stages.'

Programme of study *Pupils should be taught to:*

a   create and perform fluent sequences on the floor and using apparatus

b   include variations in level, speed and directions in their sequences.

Attainment target *Pupils should be able to demonstrate that they can:*

a   link skills, techniques and ideas and apply them appropriately, showing precision, control and fluency

b   compare and comment on skills, techniques and ideas used in own and others' work and use this understanding to improve their own performances by modifying and refining skills and techniques.

Main NC headings when considering assessment, achievement and progression

○ **Planning** – in a focused, thoughtful, safe way, thinking ahead to an intended outcome. Evidence of satisfactory planning can be seen in:

  a   good decision-making, sensible, safe judgements and good understanding of what was asked for

  b   an understanding of the elements that enhance quality, variety and contrast in 'movement'

  c   the expression of personal qualities such as optimism, enthusiasm, and a capacity for hard work in pursuit of improvement.

○ **Performing and improving performance** successfully is the main aim. In a satisfactory performance a pupil demonstrates:

  a   well-controlled, neat and accurate work, concentrating on the main feature of the task

  b   the ability to practise to improve skilfulness, performing safely

  c   whole-hearted and vigorous activity, sharing the space sensibly and unselfishly, with a concern for own and others' safety

  d   the ability to remember and repeat actions.

○ **Linking actions** – as pupils build longer, more complex sequences of linked actions in response to the stimuli, demonstrating that they are:

  a   working harder for longer, showing a clear beginning, middle and end to their sequence

  b   pursuing almost non-stop, vigorous and enjoyable action.

○ **Reflecting and evaluating** – as pupils describe what they and others have done, say what they liked about a performance, give an opinion on how it might be improved; and then make practical use of such reflection to plan again to improve.

Year 5 Gymnastic Activities Programme

Pupils should be able to:

Autumn	Spring	Summer
1 Participate and co-operate unselfishly. Aim to improve and be told you have improved.	**1** Practise enthusiastically to improve and consolidate skills.	**1** Be able to repeat movements learned previously.
2 In longer, more skilful sequences, start and finish, still, and link movements neatly to maintain flow.	**2** Experience different shapes in held positions, while travelling, and in flight.	**2** Plan appropriate use of space to respond to challenges to travel on floor and apparatus.
3 Modify initial attempts to achieve an intended result.	**3** Improve the appearance of the work with 'firm', clear shapes.	**3** Make quick decisions during non-stop travelling, finding space by looking ahead.
4 Introduce direction changes for variety and safety.	**4** Work harder for longer in almost non-stop action, in creating own planned sequences.	**4** Explore different means of rolling, taking weight on hands, balancing, running and jumping.
5 In balances, use varied parts for support, often linking the balances by rolls.	**5** Learn safe ways to land, grip, travel, balance, hang, swing.	**5** Refine and repeat longer sequences, emphasising changes of speed, effort, shape, direction or level to enhance the appearance of the work.
6 Revise safe grips on bars, boxes, benches, ropes and safe hand and arm positions while inverted on hands.	**6** Perform effectively in activities needing quick decision-making.	**6** Plan to demonstrate neat, quiet and accurate performances; to work thoughtfully; and then plan again for higher standards.
7 Practise, almost non-stop, always aware of others. 'Be found working, not waiting.'	**7** Improve quality and variety through varied shapes, levels, direction and speed.	**7** Work co-operatively with a partner, adapting favourite movement patterns to accommodate one another.
8 Maintain good posture; be physically active, using joints to their full range.	**8** Make more adventurous use of own personal and whole room, shared space, directions and levels.	**8** Demonstrate understanding through the ability to observe, copy and repeat partner's demonstrations.
9 Help self by making simple comments on own and others' performances.	**9** Sustain energetic activity by whole-hearted, vigorous activity.	**9** Be aware of and include contrasting actions for greater quality, variety and enhanced appearance.
10 Plan, practise, improve, remember and be able to repeat the longer sequences.	**10** Learn or improve simple, traditional gymnastic skills including rolls, balances, rope climbs, vaults, hand balances.	**10** Make a positive contribution within group activity.
	11 Comment on a performance and suggest ways to improve it.	**11** Analyse two performances and indicate differences in content, quality and effectiveness.

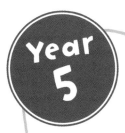

Year 5

Lesson Plan 1 • 10-15 minutes
September

At the start of the year with a new class we should be aiming to: *(a) establish a tradition of listening carefully to the teacher and making an immediate, whole-hearted, enthusiastic and vigorous response; (b) create a caring atmosphere of respect for others and self, and always moving carefully and sensibly; (c) establish a well ordered and quiet atmosphere.*

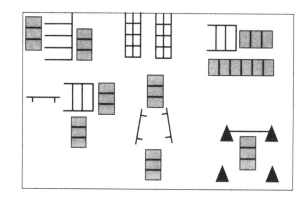

Floorwork
12–15 minutes

Legs

1   Good running is quiet and you don't follow anyone. Show me your best running and visit every part of the room, the sides, the corners, the ends and the middle.

2   When I call 'Stop!' be in a space all by yourself, well away from apparatus and other children. Stop!

3   As you run, change speed to avoid others and weave in and out of others carefully.

Body

1   Stand tall and stretched in your own space. With a three step run, show me a beautifully stretched high jump, with arms stretched to the ceiling. Do a soft 'squashy' landing with knees and ankles bending like springs, gently.

2   Look for a new space near you, and off you go again.

Arms

Travel about the room on hands and feet, very slowly. When you have lots of space around you, can you spread your body wide as you travel?

Apparatus Work
16-18 minutes

1   Travel to all parts of the room, touching floor and mats only. You can go under, over, along, across and through apparatus, but do not touch any part of it yet.

2   When I call 'Stop!' show me a clear, firm body shape on the nearest piece of apparatus. Stop!

3   Next time I call 'Stop!' show me your still, held shape on a different piece of apparatus on a different body part or parts.

4   Can you show me how you can travel, freely, on all apparatus, using hands and feet as your supports? Where possible, I would like to see you leaving your apparatus with a lively high jump and a soft, quiet, 'squashy' landing.

5   Now stay at your starting apparatus position to practise, repeat, improve and remember the following.
   a   Start and finish away from the apparatus and always be aware of where others in your group are working.
   b   Travel up to, on, along, across or around, then away from your set of apparatus.
   c   Include travelling on feet, and on hands and feet.
   d   Include a beautiful stretch at one or more points. (At start, finish, in flight, in balance.)

Final Floor Activity
2 minutes

Lift knees, ankles and arms to make your running quiet and as good as you can make it.

Teaching notes and NC guidance
Development over 4 lessons

NC elements being emphasised:

a Being physically active.
b Responding readily to instructions.
c Adopting good posture and the appropriate use of the body.

Floorwork

Legs

1 Beware of whole class, anti-clockwise running, all following all in a big circle, and common in primary schools. They need to be taught 'Run on straight lines, not curves. Do not follow anyone.'

2 The instruction 'Stop!' given two or three times, makes them run quietly, listening for the signal, and gives practice in 'responding readily to instructions'. Slow responders should be warned to smarten up, and not waste class time.

3 'Changing speed' includes running on the spot, if necessary, if there is suddenly a crowded area ahead.

Body

1 'Feel your body tension, firming up your arms, trunk and legs in flight. No limp, sagging, lazy body parts, please.'

2 A two-footed take-off is good for height, and landing with one foot after the other slows down the landing for better control.

Arms

'Spreading your body wide' will include long cartwheels, walking on hands with feet apart, travelling on hands and feet, keeping arms and legs long, straight and wide apart, bouncing along on wide hands and feet at the same time, up and down off floor.

Apparatus Work

1 An exercise in travelling to visit all parts of the room, looking out for space and avoiding impeding others. Occasionally, the teacher should call 'Stop!' to check on the quality of their spacing on the floor, with no queues or overcrowding.

2 'Stop!' once again is an attention demanding exercise to lay down and demand instant responses. Insist on an immediate response on the nearest apparatus, not some distant favourite.

3 'Stop!' again, but choose a different apparatus and a different supporting part, which requires good responding and planning.

4 Hands and feet travelling should recall the extensive repertoire from previous years. Teacher commentary gives ideas to the forgetful and acts as a stimulus to all. 'I see and like cat springs along box and benches.'

5 For final sequence, *plan* your pathway up to, on, along and away from the apparatus; your travelling actions on feet, and on hands and feet; and where your beautiful, firm stretch will take place. *Perform*, practise and repeat in a focused way to improve. *Reflect* to inform, adapt, improve and inspire your next *planned* action.

Final Floor Activity

'If I close my eyes, I should not know you are there. It should be so quiet and well controlled.'

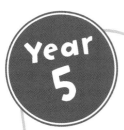

Year 5

Lesson Plan 2 • 30-35 minutes
October

Theme: *Encouraging a tradition of quiet, thoughtful, varied, and continuous work, always with an awareness of good spacing.*

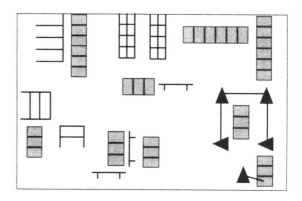

Floorwork
12—15 minutes

Legs

1 Travel from space to space in the hall, using feet only.

2 Plan to include three different actions where one is quiet and easy, one includes a direction change, and one really explodes into a vigorous movement.

Body

1 Start with your body crouched low on two feet, knees fully bent, head down to knees. With a strong lunge in one leg, stretch your body fully.

2 Can you stretch your arms strongly upwards in the lunge?

3 Bring the rear foot up beside the forward foot and curl down fully again.

4 Continue your stretching, lunging and curling in different directions with a variety of upper body stretches in the lunge position.

Arms

1 Moving slowly, quietly and continuously, can you plan a three part sequence of ways to go from feet to hands and back to feet?

2 Can you aim for variety from different body shapes, or different take-off or landing actions?

Apparatus Work
16-18 minutes

In your group places, plan how you can practise, improve and remember the following, where the emphasis is on 'Always be found working, not waiting.'

Climbing frames

As you travel, going through spaces, let different parts lead.

Ropes, mats

In addition to swinging and climbing can you show me two other actions? For example, jumping on to a swinging rope to start with; finishing with a roll on the mat; circling or hanging upside down on two ropes.

Trestles

From a starting position on the floor, well away from teammates, can you all share the apparatus and use all the surfaces? Travelling from a curl to a stretch as we did in the floorwork would be interesting.

Benches

Can you plan to include travelling, rolling and jumping? Travelling can include using hands and feet or feet only on, along or from the benches. Rolls can be from sitting, crouching or kneeling on the benches on to mats. In your explosive jumps you can use benches as springboards.

Boxes

In your continuous circuit, can you cross the cross box with legs straight? Can you include a roll along the return, low, long, box top?

Mats

Balance; roll; balance. You can roll in whichever way you prefer and your roll should be on some body part or parts which are a good starting point for your choice of roll.

Final Floor Activity
2 minutes

Run and jump long, and carry on running and jumping without stopping.

Teaching notes and NC guidance
Development over 4 lessons

NC elements being emphasised:

a   Emphasising changes of direction through gymnastic actions.
b   Making appropriate decisions quickly and planning responses.
c   Working vigorously to develop suppleness and strength, and to exercise the heart and lungs strongly.

Teaching Points

'Be found working, not waiting' is the main emphasis of this lesson and expresses the main feature of good Physical Education, namely that it will be physical. That it is educational, also, is implicit in the increasing demands now being made for planned, thoughtful and focused performance. For example, in the travelling on feet only, good planning is needed to produce three different actions, with direction changes and a change of effort, one 'quiet and easy, one exploding into vigorous movement.' Such planning and the reflection that follows are continually being emphasised as main NC requirements, second only to the action itself.

Throughout this series of lessons, demonstrate good examples of on-going performances which contain a clear starting and finishing position; quiet, thoughtful, controlled, continuous action; and good responses to the set challenges. Follow-up class reflection and evaluation can now become more specific, enhancing the quality and variety of the work. In organising the apparatus work the teacher should ensure that he or she is saying 'Please bring out your apparatus, quietly, carefully and sensibly,' in plenty of time to allow the full 16 or 18 minutes for apparatus work which is the most important part of the lesson.

After the three, or at most four sets of apparatus have been visited and worked on, the class are asked to 'Please go back to your own, number one set of apparatus.' Groups bring out and put away the same apparatus because they know where it goes. Apparatus work should be done clockwise and anti-clockwise on alternate lessons, to cover all group places every two lessons.

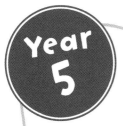

Lesson Plan 3 ● 30-35 minutes
November

Theme: *Development of variety and thoughtful, individual responses which increase the class 'repertoire' of movement.*

Floorwork
12–15 minutes

Legs

1 Can you link together several ways of travelling where your feet pass each other?

2 Remember that variety can come from different actions, in different directions, at different speeds.

Body

1 Choose some part or parts other than your feet to balance on. Stretch firmly those parts not supporting you.

2 Can you change to a new supporting part or parts?

3 Show me your choice of linking movements. Rolls are a very good 'joining up' activity.

Arms

Pretend the floorboard in front of you is a bench or a low box top. Can you travel along, across or on to this imaginary bench or box, using hands or hands and feet?

Apparatus Work
16-18 minutes

1 As you travel around freely, in and out of apparatus, without touching any, can you remind yourselves and me of the ways you chose to travel where feet pass each other?

2 When I call 'Stop!' can you show me a still, 'firm' balance on the nearest piece of apparatus? Stop!

3 When you stop in balance next time, can you show me a balance which copies or contrasts with someone near you? Stop!

4 At your varied apparatus starting places, repeat practise, improve and remember the following.

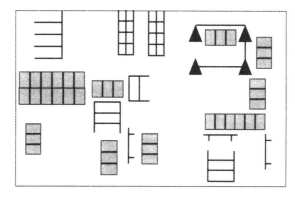

Climbing frames
Start and finish at different places on the floor and travel by changing body shapes. For example, standing and twisting to sit on; curled, stretch up to grip higher; circle around bar to balance, stretched.

Ropes
Practise the main activities that we can do on a rope. We can climb, swing, hang, circle, or a combination of two or more.

Trestles
Can you vary the body parts that lead you and show me your different travelling actions? (Lying, hanging, sliding, rolling, pulling, twisting can use many combinations of gripping or supporting parts and involve many leading parts.)

Benches
Can you start and finish in a still, balanced position on the floor away from apparatus? In between, can you plan to include flight and rolls and share all the space sensibly with others?

Low boxes, bench
Use your hands strongly to bring you on to, take you along, and help you from the apparatus. Try to include some of the activities you did in the floorwork where we had to pretend that there was a box top or a bench to work on.

Mats
Revise your sequence of balancing movements with the possibility of more adventurous links because of the mats.

Final Floor Activity
2 minutes

Follow a leader who will show you his or her ways to travel with the feet passing each other.

Teaching notes and NC guidance
Development over 4 lessons

NC elements being emphasised:

a Exploring different means of balancing and taking weight on hands.
b Making judgements of performance and suggesting ways to improve.

Floorwork

Legs

1 Feet 'pass each other' while walking, running, skipping, sliding, galloping.

2 A sequence of three different actions is long enough to be varied and interesting, and short enough to be remembered.

Body

1 Teacher commentary and good use of demonstrations will help the class repertoire in this quite difficult activity. Emphasise that 'balance' means that the body should feel like it's wobbling.

2 We do not wobble or sag lazily in the balance, but show firmness particularly in those body parts not supporting us, usually a leg or an arm. On the change to a new balance we relax into the roll, twist, lower, rock, lean linking movement between balances.

Arms

Pretending that they are working on a bench or a low box top limits the space they need and it gives good ideas for crossing from side to side; on to, along and off; twisting as you travel.

Apparatus Work

1 As well as feet passing each other, we want pupils to be passing each other, face to face, rather than all following each other, in the big anti-clockwise circle, common in primary schools.

2 Encourage balancing on parts other than feet, or feet and hands which are the most commonly seen. Praise those working hard to give a good body tension from head to toes.

3 The person with whom you choose to contrast might not even be aware that you are contrasting with him or her, as he or she relates to another. 'Contrast' is in the shape, but can be on parts supporting and level used.

Climbing frames
Remind them to keep thumbs gripping under and fingers gripping over bars for a safe, strong grip.

Ropes
Encourage and assist those who are still learning to climb by placing hands under their crossed feet on the rope to give them something to push against.

Trestles
Think about actions and the way that your body parts are supporting you. I might ask for three quite different examples.

Benches, mats
Flight can come from run along or run up to and jump from cross bench. Rolls can come after landing, and from sitting or crouch on bench.

Low box, bench
A revision of floorwork activity, done 'live'.

Mats
'More adventurous' headstand or handstand balance, rolling out balance on some other parts.

Final Floor Activity

Ask for emphasis on clear body shape as the way to make it special.

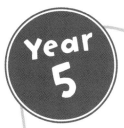

Year 5

Lesson Plan 4 • 30-35 minutes
December

Theme: *Body parts awareness and how they receive, support balance, lead into and out of movements.*

Floorwork
12—15 minutes

Legs

1   Can you run and jump high, run and jump long, using good arm and leg actions to help you at take-off, in flight, and on landing?

2   Two-footed take-offs for upward jumps and one-footed take-offs for long jumps are worth trying.

3   Arms can balance you, stretched firmly, forwards or sideways.

Body

1   Show me three bridge-like shapes, neatly linked.

2   Variety can come from using different supporting body parts – standing; upended on shoulders; or with back, front or side towards the floor.

3   To improve the look and quality of your work, stretch strongly those parts not being used to support you.

Arms

1   With your body weight on your hands, can you move your feet in different ways?

2   Can you bunny jump up and down on the spot; cartwheel to a new floorspace; jump feet to a position between hands; jump feet to a position outside hands; hand-walk to a new spot?

Apparatus Work
16-18 minutes

1   Travel freely up to, and on to, each piece of apparatus to show a still, stretched balance on each one.

2   Still using all the apparatus freely, can you plan to include?

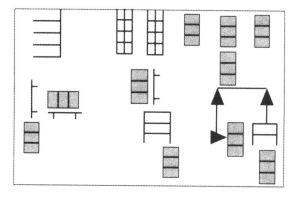

a   Travelling on the floor which is interesting because it uses parts in addition to feet.

b   Actions where the arms take all the weight.

c   A strong upwards jump.

d   A still bridge-like position.

Mats
Revise your sequence of three bridges and improve it by using different supporting parts and different levels.

Climbing frames
As you travel about the whole frame, find body parts on which you can hold a balance.

Ropes
Practise crossed foot grip on your rope. Knees are apart and rope is gripped firmly under sole of one foot and above instep of other. With arms straight, hands together and crossed foot grip, practise a small swing.

Trestles
Plan to find the body parts that can grip the apparatus as you mount on, travel along, around or under, or hold a balance.

Bench, box
Use your legs strongly to bring you on to, take you along, and to help you leave the apparatus.

Benches
Use hands and feet to support you as you zig-zag along the long bench and cross the mat. Use hands to support you as you bring both feet on to cross bench before springing off.

Final Floor Activity
2 minutes

Run and jump high; land; lower and roll sideways, curled up small, on to front; take weight on both hands.

Teaching notes and NC guidance
Development over 4 lessons

NC elements being emphasised:

a Exploring different means of jumping, and taking weight on hands, and adapting and refining these actions on the floor and on apparatus.

b Practising, adapting, improving and repeating longer and increasingly complex sequences of movement.

Floorwork

Legs

1 Short runs always into your jumps, often back and forwards in own space, to avoid impeding others.

2 Be aware of how feet can take off and land, always trying to drive hard and with strong ankles extension, and land with soft 'give' in those ankles.

3 The most obvious firm body tension is seen in the stretched arms which balance you, both in flight and on landings.

Body

1 Suggest a trio of bridge-like shapes for those slow to get started, for example: sit (bridge under bent knees); side falling on one hand and one foot; tiptoe standing with body arched.

2 Variety also comes from working at different levels, for example: high on tiptoes, medium in an arch; low, lying arched.

3 'Parts not supporting you' are usually an arm or a leg, or one of each. They should be strongly stretched into space.

Arms

1 It helps to pretend you are working on or along bench or low box top, as you vault, roll, cartwheel or do twisting bunny jumps.

2 An advanced challenge to see how many of the five tasks they can now achieve.

Apparatus Work

1 A momentary pause on each piece of apparatus, with a stretched balance on each, and, ideally, a wide range of supporting parts.

2 A sequence that uses on apparatus and floor all the work practised already on the floor, only.

3 They now stay at one place to practise and improve the following.

Mats
Weight on back of head or shoulders, plus heels, for example, are more comfortable on a mat than on the floor.

Climbing frames
As well as the usual hands and feet, try parts of hunk, behind knees or an elbow.

Ropes
Feel strong enough with hands together and feet crossed, to take one hand away as you swing, and not fall off the rope.

Trestles
Grip with hands in variety of ways; feet in a variety of ways; behind knees; at angle of elbows; under armpits.

Bench, box
An arm swing will help to induce a strong leg action on to and from apparatus.

Benches
Bunny jump, cat spring or cartwheeling actions as you zig-zag. 'Squat jump', i.e. through vault on to cross bench, with hands shoulder width apart and feet placed between hands. Spring off.

Final Floor Activity

The six activities are a good example of a 'longer and increasingly complex sequence of movements.'

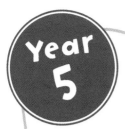

Lesson Plan 5 • 30-35 minutes
January

Theme: *Body shape awareness through which to: (a) develop an understanding of and a feeling for body shapes; (b) experience different shapes in held positions, while travelling and in flight; (c) improve the appearance of the work with 'firm' body shapes.*

Floorwork
12—15 minutes

Legs

1   Can you travel with your leg or legs sometimes stretched?

2   Can you include several actions which satisfy the task?

Body

1   Start, lying on front, back or side. Stretch your whole body from finger tips to tips of toes into a long, thin shape. Now change to a curled body where you feel that everything is tucked in, head, arms, legs.

2   Return to your original starting position, stretched out completely or move on to some other supporting parts.

Arms

1   Teach cartwheel with its wide, stretched, inverted body. Left hand on floor to side and in line with feet; right hand on floor about half a metre from left and in line with left; jump off both feet and land on right foot beyond right hand in line with hands; push with hands to stretch up, turn body and put left foot in an astride position.

2   Emphasise the left, right, left sequence along a straight line with legs as straight and high as possible.

3   Opposite, of course, if to right is preferred.

Apparatus Work
16-18 minutes

1   Use all the floor and apparatus, freely, to start with. Show me a clear body shape as you clear the lower apparatus, low boxes, benches and mats, in flight.

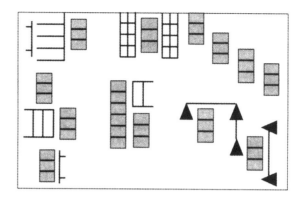

2   Show me a held position on the higher pieces of apparatus, where you have an equally clear body shape.

3   Can you walk around, practising cartwheel actions on floor, mats and benches? Emphasise the four counts of hand and foot movements and the wide stretch while inverted or partially inverted.

4   In your starting group places, practise, repeat, improve and remember the following.

Climbing frames
Start and finish on the floor. Can you twist as you travel, keeping one part fixed to twist against?

Trestles
Using apparatus and surrounding floor, can you show me some bridge-like shapes?

Box, benches
Contrast lively, stretched jumps with easy rolls.

Box, mats
Can you cross the box keeping legs straight? Can you cross the mats keeping arms and legs straight?

Mats
Revise your stretching and curling sequence and introduce more varied levels.

Ropes, bench, mats
Using two ropes, can you circle or hang upside down?

Final Floor Activity
2 minutes

Run and jump, stretched; run and jump wide; run and jump tucked, twisted or jacknifed.

Gymnastic Activities

Teaching notes and NC guidance
Development over 4 lessons

NC elements being emphasised:

a Adopting good posture and the appropriate use of the body.
b Emphasising changes of shape through gymnastic actions.

Floorwork

Legs

1 Interesting responses include full knees bend to flying stretch; hurdling, leading leg straight, steppings; hopscotch.

2 Contrasting leg actions might include lively running and jumping; soft, giving bouncing with feet together; then hopping with free leg stretched forwards.

Body

1 This can be a directed activity with the teacher slowly talking the class through it, to ensure a good start for all.

2 Other stretched positions from which to curl can be standing on one or both feet; high upended balance on shoulders; kneeling, arms stretched; headstands and handstands.

Arms

1 The 'Hand, hand, foot foot' pattern can be done on an imaginary clock face, placing hands and feet on numbers, e.g. four, two, ten and eight for a simple low angled starter.

2 The straight line target comes with practice and increasing confidence on hands.

3 A handstand practice with legs wide on the spot gives the feeling when in the middle of a cartwheel.

Apparatus Work

1 Jumping over low apparatus, including across mats, will be from one foot to other or to both after a run, or from two to two after a standing start helped by a swing with one or both arms.

2 Look out for and encourage examples of long stretch, wide stretch, curled, arched, twisted body shapes, supported on an interesting range of body parts.

3 The little walk into cartwheel provides a swing which helps. At the bench, two hands actions on the bench, two feet back on floor.

Climbing frames
Plan the pathway, floor to floor, then plan how to twist part of your body against a fixed part or parts.

Trestles
Back, front or side towards floor and apparatus, and being upended on shoulders, are possible bridges.

Box, bench
'Contrasts' can include long stretch and tight curl, and explosive jumps and gentle rolls.

Box, mats
Across box, legs can be straight as you roll, high leap, face, gate or astride vault over.

Mats
Handstands, forward rolls; bent leg to straight leg headstands now a possibility on a mat.

Ropes, bench, mats
Hold with hands at shoulder height, so that feet return to floor easily after the circle.

Final Floor Activity

A 3-metre sided triangle will bring you back to your own starting place, and not impede others.

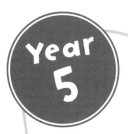

Year 5

Lesson Plan 6 • 30-35 minutes
February

Theme: *Sequences and children working harder for longer, in almost non-stop action.*

Floorwork
12—15 minutes

Legs

1 Using legs only, can you show me a triangle of movements starting and finishing at the same place on the floor, after three different actions around the triangle?

2 As always, try to start and finish, tall and still. Plan to include varied take-off and landing actions.

3 Different shapes in flight bring great variety to the work.

Body

1 Make up a short sequence of favourite balances, in your own floor space.

2 Plan to include different supporting parts for variety and interest and show a 'firm' body in balance each time.

3 Different levels give good variety when you are in your own floor space. Remember – no wobbling!

Arms

1 In a handstanding sequence can you plan to include a forward swing on to hands, a sideways swing on to hands, and a few steps on hands?

2 Throughout, keep your arms straight and head forward.

Apparatus Work
16-18 minutes

Climbing frames
Can you plan a travelling sequence which includes:
a moving hands only, then feet only;
b moving left hand and left foot, then right hand and right foot;
c weaving through spaces?

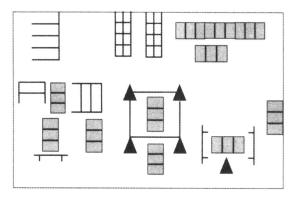

Ropes
Either try climbing, or show me a group sequence of swinging, going off one after the other and demonstrating variety in body shapes.

Trestles
In your travelling, as you all share the apparatus, use upper and lower surfaces, a variety of supporting parts, and travelling forwards, backwards, sideways, around and across.

Upturned benches
Use each of the five pieces of apparatus to demonstrate a different balance. Variety will come from varied supporting parts, levels and body shapes.

Boxes, bench
In your long circuit sequence over boxes and mats one way, and over cross bench the other way, can you:
   a make your hands important in arriving on boxes, and feet important in leaving;
   b do a vigorous spring up off the cross bench to demonstrate a different body shape to the one in front of you?

Mats
At linked trio of mats, join together two or three agilities (rolls, cartwheels, handstands, etc.). At return, single mat, can you balance, roll, balance across?

Final Floor Activity
2 minutes

Can you include examples of stillness, travelling, flight and balance in a short sequence?

Teaching notes and NC guidance
Development over 4 lessons

NC elements being emphasised:

a Exploring, selecting, developing, refining and repeating a longer series of actions, making increasingly complex sequences of movement.

b Sustaining energetic activity and understanding what happens to our bodies during exercise.

Floorwork

Legs

1 A triangle of 3–4-metre sides should not impede others and three actions provide good variety, interest and challenge.

2 Take-offs and landings in jumps, for example, can use one, both or alternate feet. The still start and finish are a good contrast to the vigorous movement.

3 Long stretched, star wide, curled tucked are very 'different'.

Body

1 'Own floor space' means on the spot, no travelling. 'Balanced' means held still, no wobbling.

2 Parts used must be a problem for balancing on, with body having to work hard to be still and under control.

3 High is often on one foot; medium can be an arch, with back, front or side to floor; low, sitting, or on elbow and heel, for example.

Arms

1 Forward swing for a still balance. Sideways swing into a cartwheel type action. Handwalking to travel a few steps.

2 Safety from straight arms and head well forward (not looking back under arms) and using just the right amount of force to swing up on to hands.

Apparatus Work

Climbing frames
Travelling, including alternating hands and feet; alternating sides of body; and weaving through spaces.

Ropes
Group swinging (after a climb), following a leader, but not following another's body shape. 'Variety' should be demonstrated.

Trestles
Group travelling and sharing with much teacher commentary on good actions and good uses of body parts seen.

Upturned benches
One of the group can set the rhythm as they move on to a piece, hold a balance for about 3 seconds, then move on to the next piece.

Boxes, bench
'Important hands' can vault, roll, twist, lever or bunny jump you on. 'Important feet' can step, jump or bounce you off.

Mats
'Agilities' mean a strong use of hands somewhere, often with inversion. For example, handstand; lower into a forward roll; stand up and finish with a cartwheel, or dive forward roll; stand and do backward roll with strong arm drive on to feet, cartwheel back to starting place.

Final Floor Activity

The mixture of calm stillness, easy travelling, vigorous leap into flight and the firm balance with non-supporting parts beautifully stretched, all add up to an interesting sequence, pleasing to performer and beholder.

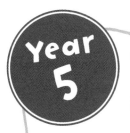
Lesson Plan 7 ● 30-35 minutes
March

Theme: *Space awareness and encouraging more adventurous and varied use of own and general space, directions and levels, both to co-operate better with others sharing the space, and to add variety and quality to our movements.*

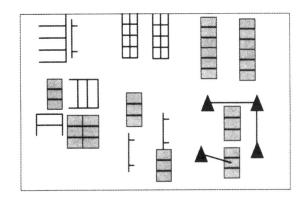

Floorwork
12–15 minutes

Legs
1   Can you make up a pattern of movements in your own space with a very small shape on the floor, such as a circle, oval or triangle?

2   Now travel, using the whole floor space and demonstrate the same shape, but on a much bigger scale, back to own place.

Body
1   Take up a position with one part of your body high. Now move to another balance with all parts close to the floor.

2   Move again and show one part very high. Continue.

Arms
1   Cartwheels travel sideways. Hand-walking travels forwards. Can you show me ways to travel backwards or diagonally, on hands only, or on hands and feet?

2   On hands and feet, remember that you can have your back or side towards the floor.

Apparatus Work
16-18 minutes

1   Using all apparatus freely, can you travel forwards on to a piece of apparatus and then travel straight along it? Can you travel sideways to the next piece, then sideways along it? Plan ahead to where you are going for such forward or sideways travelling.

2   Using hands only on the apparatus, can you lift your feet off the floor then push backwards, away from the apparatus, back on to the floor?

3   In your starting groups of fours or fives at your pieces of apparatus, can you repeat, improve and remember the following?

Climbing frames
Can you zig-zag up, head leading and zig-zag down, feet leading?

Ropes, benches
In your swinging from line to line, bench to line, or line to bench, can you make your legs work at different levels?

Trestles
Can you arrive on and leave the apparatus, using a mixture of front, back or side towards the apparatus?

Boxes, mats
Can you include low level rolls, high level jumps and at least one direction change?

Mats
a   Can you link two rolls together to show variety?
b   Sideways rolls from kneeling. One leg is stretched sideways. Roll away from the extended leg, tucking chin on to chest.

Benches (one upturned)
Balance walk along upturned bench forwards, sideways and backwards. Parts of both feet keep contact with the bench at all times. Zig-zag along return bench and mat.

Final Floor Activity
2 minutes

Run and jump into a space and continue without stopping after the jumps.

Gymnastic Activities

Teaching notes and NC guidance
Development over 4 lessons

NC elements being emphasised:

a Emphasising changes of speed through gymnastic actions.
b Making appropriate decisions quickly and planning responses.

Floorwork

Legs

1 'Pattern' means a repeating series of actions, so there must be at least two activities. Variety from actions, shapes, directions.

2 The second group of repeating actions can be different to the first, but the pathway and shape drawn must be the same.

Body

1 High level start position can be on one foot with arm upstretched. Whole body firm and still. A low balance with its element of difficulty can be on seat with arm or leg stretched and/or a leg stretched to a low level.

2 Linking movements become interesting as body weight transfers slowly, and under control. Class can be asked 'When you watch the demonstration, identify the linking movements that you liked.'

Arms

1 Easy on hands and feet. Sideways or diagonally with right arm and leg, then left arm and leg, or bouncing whole body up and from hands and feet moving sideways or backwards. Bunny jumps all ways.

2 Crabbing sideways or diagonally can have back to floor.

Apparatus Work

1 Demonstrate to extend ways of travelling sideways up to and along the apparatus. For example, slipping sideways on floor, roll sideways on mat; bounce sideways to rope, swing sideways.

2 Instead of the usual passive return of feet to floor, we push strongly to direct feet to where we want them to go.

Climbing frames
Zig-zag on one side up or weaving through spaces. Same down, or sitting weaving bar to lower bar.

Ropes, benches
Legs can hang low, be lifted to horizontal, or can grip rope above head.

Trestles
If the actions on and off are different, like the directions, this becomes an interesting and challenging activity (e.g. walk up trestle sideways; lie on plank and pull along backwards; or do forward circle over metal pole).

Boxes, mats
If the low level rolls along mats are slow and smooth and the high jumps are extremely vigorous, these contrasts, together with a change of direction, make up a good sequence.

Mats
a Forwards, backwards; hands together, hands one in front of other; both hands, no hands; long dive roll, small, curled up roll.
b A teacher directed activity, helped by one of many pupils who do it well straight away.

Benches
Feel for bench in the balance, then foot down on top. Do not look down. Moving foot runs alongside balance bar.

Final Floor Activity

Run/jump adjusted and variable to let you land in a good space, safely, not impeding others.

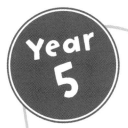

Lesson Plan 8 • 30-35 minutes
April

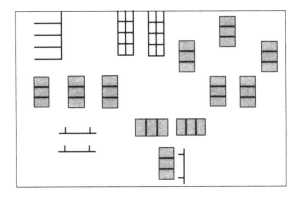

Theme: *Direct teaching of simple, traditional gymnastic skills which are part of our PE heritage – most children enjoy the stimulus of a direct challenge to their skilfulness.*

Floorwork
12—15 minutes

Legs

1 Skip jumping on the spot, with good stretch of whole body in the air, particularly the ankle joints.

2 Three skip jumps followed by a tuck jump where knees are pulled up as high as possible.

3 Four skip jumps followed by jumping feet astride and together, twice.

Body

Ski swings. Feet slightly apart. Swing both arms forwards/upwards above head. Swing arms down past sides, then up above head to high stretch. Long arm swing down and back, with full knee bend; swing arms upwards and knees stretch; long arm swing down and back, with full knee bend; swing arms upwards and knees stretch; lower arms and repeat.

Arms

Elbow balance, with hands only on floor. Crouched position with feet apart, place hands under shoulders. Bend elbows slightly to place them inside and under knees. Tilt body forwards slowly, from feet on to hands, until toes come off floor, and you are balancing on hands only.

Apparatus Work
16-18 minutes

Mats
a Forwards roll; stand up with one foot crossed behind the other; twist the body half around to side of rear foot; finish with a backward roll.

b Lie on back, curled small, hands clasped under knees. Roll to left to right, then try a roll completely over to finish on back again.

Climbing frames
a Travel vertically up, diagonally down.

b With a partner, start at opposite bottom corners. Climb to top corner and come down diagonally, meeting and passing at the centre.

Ropes
a Swing with hands gripping together and crossed foot grip. As you swing, can you take one hand off to prove a good foot grip?

b Rope climbing, using three hand movements to every lift and grip of the feet. One hand up and grip. Other hand up and grip. First hand up and grip next to second hand. Now pull both legs up and grip with crossed feet. 'Hand, hand, hands together, feet up.'

Long box, cross bench
Catspring hands and feet on to near end of long box. Either cartwheel, roll or bunny jump along and from the box. At cross bench, either face vault across on both hands, like bunny jumping, or place hands on bench and astride vault, feet on to bench outside hands. Stand up and jump off.

Mats
Bent legs headstand.

Upturned benches
Balance walk forwards.

Final Floor Activity
2 minutes

Can you plan four groups of four skip jumping activities that are all different?

Teaching notes and NC guidance
Development over 4 lessons

Gym | Year 5 | Lesson 8

NC elements being emphasised:

a   Developing skill by exploring and making up activities.
b   Trying hard to consolidate performances.

Floorwork

Legs

1   Good ankle joint activity, with full strong stretch, is essential for a good, high upwards spring, just as the 'give' in the ankles makes the landing soft and quiet without any jarring.

2   Try to feel your steady rhythm, counting in fours to yourself. A good, fully tucked jump, is a quick, dynamic movement, for which 'trying hard' is necessary.

3   'Feet together, 3, 4; out and in, 3, 4.'

Body

The swinging here is a feature of much of our gymnastic activities and is an excellent aid to all kinds of movement, including jumps, handstands, and a one arm swing into a turn as you jump from a box, for example.

Arms

Rise up on to tiptoes and lean your shoulders forwards to tilt on to hands. Hands should be pointing forwards with fingers spread.

Apparatus Work

Mats

Chin on chest forwards, heels near to seat to finish with one push only with hands. Hands by ears, thumbs in, going backwards, and strong arm push (thumbs in, still) to land on feet, not knees.

Climbing frames

Keep thumbs gripping under bar, fingers gripping over bar for a safe, strong, reliable grip.

Ropes

The climbing song: 'Hands one, two, hands together, feet up.' Legs pull up with hands together is important. Separate hands mean only upper hand is effective.

Long box, cross bench

Bunny jumps, rolls or cartwheels represent the degrees of difficulty, in that order. At cross bench, hands on and feet jumped on to bench astride hands is the first stage of the astride vault.

Mats

Bent legs headstand is the easiest 'upended' balance to hold with its triangle base and low centre of gravity. You can go into it from elbow balance.

Upturned benches

Do not look down. Feel for the side of the bar, then feel for the surface where you are to put down your foot, before committing your weight to it. Arms are stretched out to side for balance.

Final Floor Activity

Can you plan four groups of four skip jumping activities that are all different? 'Different' can also include jumps where one foot stays under you and the other reaches out to touch floor at side or front.

Year 5

Lesson Plan 9 • 30-35 minutes
May

Theme: *Travelling and the many natural body activities and movements which can be experienced, repeated, and improved in a Gymnastic Activities lesson.*

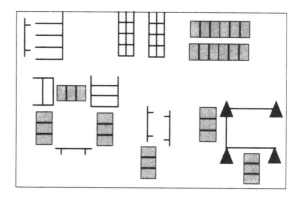

Floorwork
12–15 minutes

Legs

1 Can you walk, run, jump and land and carry on without stopping?

2 Plan to make your non-stop travelling fit the spaces you are using. Sometimes your walk and run will be very short and sometimes they can spread themselves, when you have room.

Body

1 Can you travel by changing from a fully stretched to a tightly curled shape, using different supporting body parts?

2 Your travelling will look more interesting if you change levels.

3 Lunge to crouch on feet; curled to stretched on one side; rolls from stretched, back or front lying; are some of the many possibilities.

Arms

1 Can you travel, very slowly, on hands and feet?

2 Cartwheels, handwalks, handstands down with a twist can all be 'travelling', with the emphasis on hands.

3 Strong work on hands and feet usually means straight arms and legs. Hands then feet; one side then the other; bounce up off floor at same time; travelling 'bunny jumps'.

Apparatus Work
16-18 minutes

1 Using feet only, can you travel, non-stop, to all parts of the room, without touching any apparatus other than floor and mats?

2 On floor and all apparatus, freely, can you plan ways to travel by changing from a stretched to a curled body shape? Your curled shapes can sometimes take you into a roll to travel to your next stretch.

3 Stay at your starting group places to practise, improve and remember the following.

Climbing frames
Partners, one leading, one following. Travel, going from stretches to curls.

Mats
Including a roll somewhere, can you travel along the two mats?

Bench, inverted bench
Use hands and feet to travel along one bench. Show me your different balancing travelling actions along the upturned bench.

Ropes, bench
Practise your good hand and foot grips as you swing from bench back to bench. Climbers, can you do three hand travels to every lift of your feet? One, two, hands together, feet up.

Trestles
Can you travel by bringing hands and feet near to each other, then taking them apart.

Boxes, bench
Can you plan to show me a set of contrasting travelling actions and movements? Smooth rolls; explosive jumps; weight on hands travels; twists, curls and stretches.

Final Floor Activity
2 minutes

Show a partner ways to travel, using legs only, but not including walking, running or jumping.

Teaching notes and NC guidance
Development over 4 lessons

NC elements being emphasised:

a Practising, adapting, improving and repeating longer and increasingly complex sequences of movement.
b Making judgements of performance and suggesting ways to make improvements.

Floorwork

Legs

1 Without a still start and finish, the travelling has to continue almost non-stop. This needs quick decision making as they look ahead for space, and adjust to include the three actions set.

2 Landing from the jump will be on one foot to help the change to walking. Often, the landing from the jump is near a wall, corner or busy space, and an instant direction change is needed.

Body

1 A short, directed routine of two or three movements, explained by the teacher, helps to get the whole class into action quickly.

2 After the directed start they will gradually, week by week, progress on to adding in their own ideas.

3 In a lunge, legs are spread wide, with front knee well bent, other leg straight to rear. Body leans forward over front leg with arms upstretched above head.

Arms

1 Slow travel on hands and feet, rather than quick scampering, means much harder work for the slow, neat actions.

2 Whether cartwheeling or handwalking, straight arms are needed for a safe, strong support, with the head looking forwards.

3 Travelling on all fours is a strong activity if arms and legs are wide or close, and straight. 'How high an arch can you make with arms and legs close? How low an arch without collapsing?'

Apparatus Work

1 Once again, non-stop travelling involves individuals in looking and planning ahead to negotiate apparatus, without touching it, and it involves the whole class in sensible travel, sharing well.

2 Travel by going from stretch to curl, usually by hands and feet closing and parting, is possible on all parts of all apparatus.

Climbing frames
'A' travels and stops. 'B' catches up. Much hands alone travelling to stretch, then feet curling to catch up.

Mats
Handstand, roll. Cartwheel, roll. Jump and land, roll. Bent leg headstand, tuck head on to chest, roll.

Bench, inverted bench
Balance walk forwards, backwards, sideways or cat walk with both hands and feet holding bench.

Ropes, bench
In swinging from bench back to bench, start with a strong upwards backward jump to give you, like a pendulum, plenty of swing to bring you back to bench.

Trestles
Hands then feet travel along, under, around, across, again with hands moving alone, then feet moving alone.

Boxes, bench
Non-stop, but with variety in the actions and the effort used.

Final Floor Activity

Hopscotch, bounce, skip, hop, slip sideways, plus many country dance steps, if known.

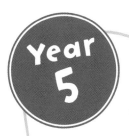

Year 5
Lesson Plan 10 • 30-35 minutes
June

Theme: *Dynamics. (a) Time and its varied use in completing actions. Slowly, quickly, slowing down, speeding up, a sudden explosive movement; (b) Flow and the variety of control being applied. From slow, flowing controlled at all times; to flat out vigorous; to linked up, with stops in between each move.*

Floorwork
12–15 minutes

Legs

1   Show me your best running, weaving in and out of others. Run at slow to medium speeds when near others. Run quickly when you have lots of space.

2   Run and jump and keep on running immediately. Then run, jump and land and be perfectly still; and controlled on landing. Can you feel the difference in these two sets of actions?

Body

1   From a standing position, can you sit down and roll back slowly and smoothly on to shoulders and hands? Then, equally smoothly, can you roll back on to your feet?

2   Repeat the whole movement, but plan to add on a quick stretch upwards of legs while on shoulders to end the backward movement, and a quick stretch up of arms to end the forward movement.

Arms

As you travel about the room, going from feet to hands and back to feet again, can you plan to demonstrate contrasting movements with some vigorous and strong, and some that are flowing and 'easy'?

Apparatus Work
16-18 minutes

1   Run all around the room, 'easy', steady, speed, touching floor and mats only.

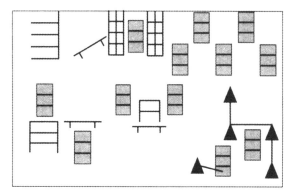

2   Now run to all parts of the room and show me a vigorous action that brings you on to a piece of apparatus, or takes you across it.

3   At your different group starting positions can you practise, repeat, improve and remember the following?

Climbing frames
From different starting places on the floor, travel smoothly and continuously before finishing on the floor.

Ropes
a   Revise swinging with strong crossed foot action, trying to take one hand off to prove a good foot grip.
b   Revise climbing, as in last month's lesson, emphasising three hand moves to every move of legs.

Mats
Revise the rocking and stretching from the floorwork, going from standing to sitting to inverted shoulder balance.

Trestles
As a group, stay on and share all the apparatus and show me a variety of actions.

Box, bench
Accelerate into an explosive high jump from the cross bench. In contrast, show me a slower, more controlled way of travelling along.

Bench, box
Including floor and apparatus, show me a sequence which uses feet to hands and back to feet activities.

Final Floor Activity
2 minutes

Can you sometimes run on the spot; at a steady rhythm; accelerate?

Teaching notes and NC guidance
Development over 4 lessons

NC requirements being emphasised:

a Emphasising changes of speed and effort through gymnastic actions.

b Exploring different means of rolling, jumping and taking weight on hands, and practising and refining these actions on the floor and on apparatus.

Floorwork

Legs

1 'Weaving in and out of others' means that there will be no following one behind the other, as in the commonplace, anti-clockwise running, all in a big circle, going the same way.

2 Checking the movement alternates with keeping it flowing. A still start, a flowing movement and a checked movement with a still, controlled finish is a way of presenting this pattern.

Body

1 Hands swing forwards as you lower to balance you, then hands are placed besides shoulders, thumbs in, hands pointing forwards, on the shoulder balance. Hands push you forwards strongly in swing up.

2 The quick upward stretch of legs while inverted will be an attractive contrast to the slow lowering that preceded it.

Arms

The kick up to handstand is a strong, vigorous movement and can contrast with the gentle return of feet back to floor. Easy, slow travel on feet and hands can contrast with the dynamic bounce off floor by hands and feet at the same time.

Apparatus Work

1 'Feel ... your rhythm; feel ... your rhythm; 1, 2, 3, 4.' Non-stop, easy jogging with heels and hands not as high as in high quality running, feeling your own easy 'cruising' speed.

2 Now there will be acceleration, leading to the mount on to, or the crossing of, the apparatus, whether with feet or hands being used to support you as you arrive on, or cross the apparatus.

Climbing frames
This virtually non-stop travelling will need the co-operation of all concerned.

Ropes
a Hands are one on top of other and feet are one on top of other (sole over instep), working as one for a secure grip.

b Emphasise that hands must be together at the time legs are lifted, the most difficult part.

Mats
Finish on one leg, or with feet crossed.

Trestles
Seldom needs an approach from the floor, and a group can stay on for quite long periods, using all surfaces.

Box, bench
The return activity set-up means no queuing and the group can follow, non-stop, as they circulate, demonstrating the contrasts of speed.

Bench, box
Feet to hands back to feet includes rolls along and from apparatus on to mats; bunny jump actions on to, along and from apparatus; vaults across apparatus.

Final Floor Activity

When space is limited, run on spot. When space is reasonable, run steady. With plenty of room, accelerate.

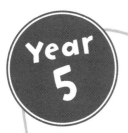

Lesson Plan 11 • 30-35 minutes
July

Theme: *Partner work to provide new experiences through adapting favourite movement patterns to accommodate another. Pleasurable social relationships are being developed.*

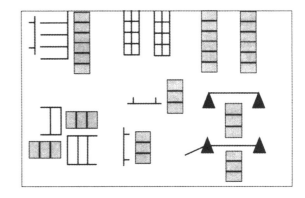

Floorwork
12–15 minutes

Legs

1 Follow your leader who will show you some lively, warming-up activities, using legs.

2 On the spot, facing each other now, the new leader will demonstrate variations of skip jumping (e.g. feet together; feet apart; feet parting and closing; feet parting and crossing; four, then turn to right, four, then turn to front).

Body

Partner 'A' holds various bridge-like shapes and 'B' has to wind in, out, through or over, without touching 'A'. Change.

Arms

First partner performs a movement while weight is on hands or hands and feet. Other partner copies this one movement and adds another. This continues until a 4–6 part sequence has been formed.

Apparatus work
16-18 minutes

1 Using all the floor space freely, follow your leader, whose actions are designed to take you around, across, through or astride the apparatus, but touching only the floor and the mats.

2 New leader, can you hold a bridge-like shape on apparatus, or apparatus and floor, while your partner weaves under, through or over you?

3 At your starting apparatus places, repeat, practise, improve and remember the following.

Climbing frames

Start at opposite bottom corners. Climb vertically to top corner. Descend diagonally, passing in the centre, to finish in your partner's place.

Ropes, bench, mats

a Climb one rope, cross to second rope, descend one after the other.

b Share one rope where leader swings from mat to bench, etc., then passes rope to partner with a swing for him or her to follow.

Bench, inverted bench, trestle, mats

Going from apparatus to apparatus, show your partner a favourite balance. Space permitting, your partner might try to mirror you.

Boxes, mats

Starting at opposite sides, build up to a matching sequence with the emphasis on clear body shapes.

Trestles

Start at opposite ends of the apparatus. Approach, meet, pass and finish in your partner's place.

Mats

One partner lies in various shapes on the mat and other partner has to jump over, showing a matching shape. Change duties.

Final Floor Activity
2 minutes

Facing each other, one partner leads in a simple jumping routine on the spot. Groups of four jumps are recommended.

Teaching notes and NC guidance
Development over 4 lessons

NC elements being emphasised:

a Working safely, alone and with others.
b Making appropriate decisions quickly and planning their responses.
c Making judgements of performance and suggesting ways to improve.

Floorwork

Legs

1 'Lively' infers vigorous, powerful, whole-hearted, strong.

2 Establish a joint rhythm which can almost be felt and heard, so that your duo could almost keep going with eyes shut. It is a fairly slow rhythm if there is a dynamic drive from strong ankles giving a high lift.

Body

Still partner can make three bridges, one after the other, to give travelling partner some variety, from an easy high bridge on both feet with body angled forwards, down to a difficult low level arch, say, on elbows and knees.

Arms

This gradual build-up activity is most popular with all pupils. Partners need to make considerate allowance for each other, only showing something within other partner's capability. The build-up extends over the four or five week period of this lesson, and they don't need to do all in one lesson.

Apparatus Work

1 Practise following at 2 metres behind leader to see easily the actions, uses of body parts, shapes and directions being offered.

2 The weaving of the floorwork transfers to apparatus, or apparatus and floor, as they circulate to each apparatus in turn. A high arch with back or front towards apparatus is a quick method.

Climbing frames
Starting on opposite sides will let you mirror each other with hands, feet and bodies moving in unison.

Ropes, bench
Climb half way, then carefully cross to next rope. In the swings, remember to jump up and back at start of swing to produce a big pendulum action for a long enough swing.

Benches, trestle
Contrasting supporting parts and shapes would be a good challenge as they circulate, balancing alternately.

Boxes, mats
Agree the actions, then decide on body shapes to be emphasised and any direction changes. Will there be a spectacular change of speed or effort at some point?

Trestles
Passing on a plank is easy with one sitting or crouching, one going over. Passing on a metal pole is very difficult, with one above and one below.

Mats
Matching tucked, wide star, long stretched, arched or twisted shapes.

Final Floor Activity

Simple foot movements (together, parting and closing, turning to face each wall) can be enhanced by the addition of matching arm movements (swinging to side, front or above head).

Dance

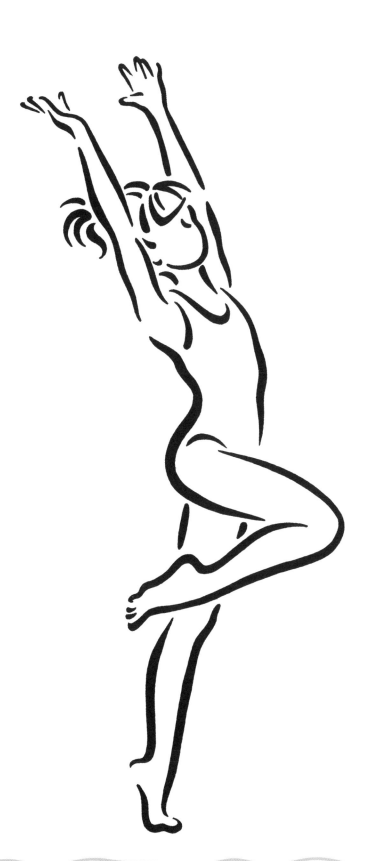

The Aims of Dance

Education has been described as the 'structuring of experiences in such a way as to bring about an increase in human capacity.' Dance aims to increase human capacity under the following headings:

1 **Physical development**. We focus on body action to develop skilful, well-controlled, versatile movement. We want our pupils to move well, looking poised and confident. The vigorous actions in dance also promote healthy physical development, fitness and strength.

2 **Knowledge and understanding**. Pupils learn and understand through the combination of physical activity (with its doing, feeling and experiencing of movement) and the mental processes of decision-making, as they plan, refine, evaluate and then plan again for improvement.

3 **Enjoyment**. Dance is fun and an interesting, sociable, enjoyable physical activity. In addition to the perspiration and deep breathing which the vigorous physical activity inspires, there should be smiling faces expressing enjoyment. When asked why they like something, pupils' first answer is usually 'It's fun!' It is hoped that enjoyable, sociable and physical activity experienced regularly at school in dance and other physical education lessons, can have an influence on pupils' eventual choice of lifestyle, long after they have left school. We want them to understand that regular physical activity makes you look and feel better, and helps to make you feel relaxed, calm and fit.

4 **Confidence and self-esteem**. Particularly at primary school, a good physical education that recognises and praises achievement can enhance an individual's regard for him or herself, and help to improve confidence and self-esteem. Dance lessons are extremely visual and offer many opportunities to see improvement, success and creativity; demonstrating these admirable achievements to others; and helping pupils feel good about themselves.

5 **Social development**. Friendly, co-operative social relationships are part of most dance lessons. Achievement, particularly in the 'dance climax' part of the lesson, is usually shared with a partner or a small group. Pupils also share space sensibly with others; take turns at working; demonstrate to, and watch demonstrations by, others; and make appreciative, helpful comments to demonstrators and partners.

6 **Creativity**. It has been said that 'if you have never created something, you have never experienced satisfaction.' Dance is a most satisfying activity, regularly challenging pupils to plan and present something original. Opportunities abound for an appreciative teacher to say 'Thank you for your demonstration and your own, original way of doing the movements.'

7 **Expression and communication**. In dance we communicate through the expression in movement of the feelings or the action. We use, for example, stamping feet to express anger; we skip, punch the air or clap hands to show happiness; we swagger, head held high, to express self-assurance. Similarly, we create simple characters and stories by expressing them through movements associated with them. The old or young; machine or leaves; puppet, animal or circus clown, can all be expressed through their particular way of moving.

8 **Artistic and aesthetic appreciation**. Gaining knowledge and understanding of the quality-enhancing elements of movement is a particular aim of dance. Such understanding of quality, variety and contrast in the use of body action, shape, direction, size, speed and force, is a major contributor to appreciation of good movement. We want our pupils to understand what is good about good movement.

Stimuli as Starting Points with Which to Inspire Dance Action

Stimuli are used to gain the interest of the class, provide a focus for their attention, get them into the action quickly, and inspire in them a desire for movement.

A dance stimulus is something you:

○ **enjoy doing**, such as natural actions. Pupils will immediately start to walk, run, jump, skip, hop, bounce or gallop, whether accompanied by music, percussion, following the teacher/leader, or responding to an enthusiastic teacher calling out the actions.

○ **can hear**. Sounds that stimulate movement include:

a medium to quick tempo music, including folk dance music

b percussion instruments – tambourine, drum, cymbal, clappers

c body contact sounds – clapping hands, stamping feet, slapping body, clicking fingers

d rhythmically chanted phrases, words, place names or actions which can be shortened or elongated to inspire and accompany actions

e vocal sounds to accompany actions, on the spot and travelling as in 'toom, toom, toom' marching; 'boomp, boomp, boomp' bouncing; and 'tick, tock, tick, tock' slow stepping

f action songs, chanted rhymes and nursery rhymes.

○ **can see or imagine**. Objects like a leaf, branch, balloon, ball, bubble, puppet, rag doll, firework, can all be used to suggest movement ideas to children. Use of imagery and imagination helps to communicate what we are trying to express more clearly. 'Can you creep softly and slowly, as if you did not want to be heard, coming home late?'

○ **have seen on a visit, on television, or in a photograph**. Of particular interest to pupils are:

a zoo animals – penguins. elephants, dolphins, monkeys

b circus performers – jugglers, clowns, trapeze artists, acrobats, tightrope walkers

c seaside play – swimming, paddling, making sandcastles, plus movements of the waves

d children's playground activities – climbing, swinging, sea-saw, throwing and catching, skipping, circling on a roundabout.

○ **experience seasonally** – spring and growth, summer holidays, autumn and harvest, winter snow and frost, Guy Fawkes' Night, Halloween, Christmas toys, circus and pantomime, Easter eggs.

○ **consider newsworthy or of human interest** – Olympic Games, extremes of weather, newly arrived pupils, hobbies, family, friendship, approaching holidays.

Whatever the starting point, the teacher must convert it into the language of movement. Children cannot 'be' leaves, but they can 'Travel on tip toes with light, floating movements, tilting and turning slowly.' They cannot 'be' clowns, but they can 'Do a funny walk on heels, spin round with one leg high, fall down slowly, bounce up and repeat.' They cannot 'be' machines, but they can 'Try pushing down actions, like corks into bottles, on the spot, turning or moving along, as on an assembly line.'

The Creative Dance Lesson Plan

Warming up Activities which start the lesson are important because they can create an attentive, co-operative, industrious and thoughtful start to the lesson, put the class in the mood for dance, and encourage them to move with good body poise and tension, sharing the floor unselfishly. The activities need to be simple enough to get the whole class working, almost immediately, often by following the teacher who, ideally, is a stimulating **'purveyor of action'** enthusiastically leading the whole class, often by example, into wholehearted participation in simple activities which need little explanation. Some form of travelling, using the feet, is often the warming-up activity, with a specific way of moving being asked for. It might be to show better use of space, greater variety, greater control, good poise and body tension, or simply an enthusiastic use of all the body parts to warm up.

The Movement Skills Training middle part of the lesson is used to teach and develop the movement skills and patterns that are to be used in the new dance. Here, the teacher is an **educator**, informing, challenging, questioning, using demonstrations and sometimes direct teaching.

a   Kneel down and curl to your smallest shape. Show me how you can start to grow, very slowly. Are you starting with your back, head, shoulders, elbows or arms? Show me clearly how you rise to a full, wide stretch position.

b   If gesturing is like speaking with your body's movement, how might your body gesture say 'I am angry'? Stamp feet, clench fists, punch the air, jump up and down heavily.

c   How are bubbles (made by teacher and pupils) moving? Where are they going? Floating gently, gliding smoothly, soaring from low to higher, sinking slowly.

The creating and performing Dance Climax of the lesson is the most important part and must not be missed out or rushed. If necessary, earlier parts of the lesson should be reduced. Here the teacher is a **coach**, helping and guiding the pupils as they work at their creation, moving round to all parts of the room to advise, encourage, enthuse, praise and, eventually, demonstrate.

a   Slowly, start to grow and show me which parts are leading as you rise to your full, wide flower shape in our 'Spring Dance'. You might even twist your flower shape to look at the sun.

b   Find a partner for our 'Gestures' dance and decide who is asking a favour by gesturing with body actions to say 'Please! I'm desperate! I need it! I must have it!' The other partner's body actions are saying 'Never! You must be joking! Go away!' When we look at demonstrations later, we will decide who the most expressive winners are.

c   For our 'Bubbles dance', I will say the four actions that are to be practised – floating gently, gliding smoothly, soaring, sinking slowly, and you will show me how you have planned to dance them.

Depending on its complexity, a dance lesson will be repeated three or four times to allow sufficient time for repetition, practice and improvement to take place, and a satisfactory performance to be achieved and presented.

It has been said that 'dance is all about making, remembering and repeating patterns.' Whether we are performing a created dance or an existing folk dance, there will still be a still start and finish, and an arrangement of repeated parts within.

The Traditional Folk Dance Lesson Plan – 30 minutes

Warming-up activities – 5 minutes

These varied steps can relate to the new figures to be taught, or they can be travelling steps or steps on the spot of any kind, to stimulate quick, easy enjoyable action to put the class in the mood for dance. The warm-up can be done alone or with a partner. As well as inspiring action, the teacher establishes high standards of neat footwork and good, safe, unselfish sharing of space. For example, 'Skip by yourself, to visit all parts of the room, keeping in time with the music.' 'When drum sounds twice, join hands with the nearest person and dance together.' 'When drum sounds once, dance by yourself again.'

Teach figures of new dance – 14 minutes

Teaching is easier in a big circle formation where everyone can see and copy the teacher. Often, all can perform the whole dance together, slowly and carefully, figure by figure, practising it to the teacher's voice, then doing it at the correct speed. The teacher's non-stop vocal accompaniment, along with the actions, serves to remind the class of the actions and keeps them moving at the correct speed. For example, 'Everyone ready... Skip to the centre, 2, 3, turn on 4; back to places, 2, 3, arrive on 4. Boys to centre, 2, 3, turn on 4; back to places, 2, 3, there on 4. Girls to centre, 2, 3, turn on 4; back to places, 2, 3, hands joined on 4. All circle left, 2, 3, 4, 5, 6, back the other way; circle right, 2, 3, 4, 5, 6, ready to start again.'

Teaching in sets of two, three, four or more couples is more difficult because the sets are separate, with someone's back to the teacher. Each leading couple in turn will be taken slowly through the figures, then walking, then dancing to the music or the teacher's vocal accompaniment.

Teach the new dance – 7 minutes

Ideally, the new dance will be performed without stopping, helped by early reminders to the next dancers from the teacher's continuous vocal accompaniment. It is sometimes necessary to stop the music after each dancing couple has completed the dance, because of problems experienced by some of the dancers. The new couples are put in position, the music is re-started, and they do the dance once again.

Revise a favourite dance – 4 minutes

This last dance, often chosen by pupils, should be a contrast to the lesson's new dance, for variety. A lively circle dance, with all dancing non-stop, can be contrasted with a set dance where only one or two of the four couples are dancing at a time.

Teaching Dance With 'Pace'

High on the list of accolades for an excellent dance lesson is the comment that 'it had excellent pace' and moved along, almost non-stop, from start to finish. Lesson pace is determined by the way that each of the several skills making up the whole lesson is taught. For example:

1   **Quickly into action**. Using few words, explain the skill clearly and challenge the class to begin. 'Show me your best stepping, in time with the music. Begin!' This near-instant start is helped if the teacher joins in and works enthusiastically with them.

2   **Emphasise the main teaching points, one at a time, while class is working**. The class all need to be working quietly if the teacher is to be heard. 'Visit all parts of the room – sides, ends and corners, as well as the middle.' 'Travel along straight lines, never following anyone.' (Primary school pupils always travel in a big anti-clockwise circle, all following one another, unless taught otherwise.)

3   **Identify and praise good work while the class is working**. The class teacher does not say 'well done' without being specific and explaining what is praiseworthy. Comments are heard by all and remind the class of key points. 'Well done, Emily. Your tip toe stepping is lively and neat.' 'Liam, you keep finding good spaces to travel through. Well done.'

4   **Teach for individual improvement, while the class is working**. 'Ben, swing arms and legs with more determination, please.' 'Lucy, use your eyes each time you change direction to see where the best space is.'

5   **Use a demonstration, briefly,** to show good quality, or a good example of what is expected and worth copying. 'Stop, please, and watch Olivia, Michael, James and Ravinder step out firmly with neat, quiet footwork, never following anyone.' 'Stop and watch how Chloe is mixing bent, straight and swinging leg actions for variety.'

6   **Very occasionally, to avoid using too much activity time, a short demonstration is followed by comments from observers**. 'Half of the class will watch the other half. Look out for and tell me whose stepping is neat, lively and always well spaced. Tell me if someone impresses you for any other reason.' The class watch for about 12 seconds and three or four comments are listened to. For example: 'James is mixing tiny steps with big ones.' 'Maisie is stepping with feet passing each other, then with feet wide apart.' Halves of the class change over and repeat the demonstrations with comments.

7   **Thanks are given to all the performers and to those who made helpful, friendly comments**. Further practice takes place with reminders of the good things seen and commented on.

A Pattern for Looking at and Developing Dance Movement

To avoid confusing him or herself and the class, the teacher will be thinking about, looking for and talking about one element within dance at a time. If, in the early stages of a lesson's development, the teacher is only looking for the actions and how the body parts concerned are performing them, there is some hope for progress and improvement. If, on the other hand, the teacher is exhorting the class to think about 'your spacing, actions, shape, speed – and what about some direction changes?', all at the same time, then confusion will be the only outcome.

Stage 1 The Body

What is the pupil doing?

1   **Actions**   travelling, jumping, turning, rolling, balancing, gesturing, rising, falling, etc..

2   **Body parts important**   legs, feet, hands, shoulders, head, etc..

3   **Body shape**   stretched, curled, wide. twisted, arched.

Stage 2 The Space

Where is the pupil doing it?

1   **Directions**   forwards, backwards, sideways.

2   **Level**   high, medium, low.

3   **Size**   own, little, personal space; whole room, large general space shared with others.

CHILD

DANCING

Stage 3 The Quality

How is the pupil doing it?

1   **Weight or effort**   firm, gentle, vigorous, light, heavy.

2   **Time or speed**   sudden, fast, slow, speeding up, slowing down, explosive.

Stage 4 The Relationships

With whom is the pupil doing it?

1   **Alone**   but always conscious of sharing space with others.

2   **Teacher**   near, following, mirroring, in circle with, away from, towards.

3   **Partner**   leading, following, meeting, parting, mirroring, copying, making contact with.

4   **Group**   circle, part of class for a demonstration

Headings When Considering a Pupil's Achievement and Progress Through Dance

Physical fitness

Strong, often prolonged physical activity, inspired by vigorous leg action, helps to promote normal, healthy growth and physical development. Lively leg action in dance also stimulates strong heart and lungs activity, leading to improved stamina.

Physical skill and versatility

Body management and self-control, called for in challenging situations, develops skill in natural actions such as travelling, jumping and landing, balancing, rolling, turning, rising and falling. When body management and self-control are good, there is an impression of poised, confident, versatile, safe movement.

Feeling valued and self-confident

Using their imagination, being creative, planning something original, and then sharing it with others, can develop and improve pupils' self confidence and self-esteem, particularly when the teacher and the class warmly and enthusiastically express their appreciation for the achievement. We want our dancers, eventually, to exude confidence and enthusiasm.

Expressing themselves

Using the body as an instrument of expression, and another way to communicate, pupils can express emotions, inner feelings, moods, convey ideas, and even create simple characters and stories. For many, this is a totally different, potentially eloquent outlet for expressing feeling as they stamp the work with their own personality.

Learning to develop friendly, co-operative, working relationships with others

Dance is the most sociable of physical education's activities. Working in pairs and groups; sharing space; taking turns; demonstrating and being demonstrated to; and appreciating and being appreciated by others, encourages desirable, enjoyable, co-operative social relationships.

Believing in the value of participation in physical activity

We want pupils to look and feel better after exercise, and believe that physical activity is enjoyable, and an essential antidote to the increasingly sedentary, inactive lifestyle of many people.

Becoming more competent, knowledgeable performers and spectators

Dance education develops an appreciation of the aesthetic and expressive elements within dance – variety and contrast in actions, shape, direction and level, speed, and degree of force.

National Curriculum Requirements for Dance – Key Stage 2: the Main Features

Programme of study Pupils should be taught to:

a create and perform dances using a range of movement patterns, including those from different times and cultures

b respond to a range of stimuli and accompaniment.

Attainment target Pupils should be able to demonstrate that they can:

a link skills, techniques and ideas and apply them accurately and appropriately, showing precision, control and fluency

b compare and comment on skills, techniques and ideas used in others' work, and use this understanding to improve their own performance by modifying and refining skills and techniques.

Main NC headings when considering progression and expectation

Planning – This provides the focus and the concentrated thinking necessary for an accurate performance. Where standards of planning are satisfactory, there is evidence of:

a the ability to think ahead, visualising what you want to achieve

b good decision-making, selecting the most appropriate choices

c a good understanding of what was asked forand of quality, variety and contrast

d an unselfish willingness to listen to others' views and adapt own performance correspondingly.

Performing and improving performance – This is always the most important feature of a lesson. We are fortunate that the visual nature of Physical Education enables pupils' achievement to be easily seen, shared and judged. Where standards in performing are satisfactory, there is evidence of:

a successful, safe outcomes in neat, accurate, 'correct' performances

b consistency, and the ability to repeat and remember

c economy of effort and making everything look 'easy'

d adaptability, making sudden adjustments as required.

Linking actions – With a view to getting pupils working harder for longer, which is a main aim for Physical Education teaching, encourage them to pursue near-continuous, vigorous and enjoyable action, expressed ideally in deep breathing, perspiration and smiling faces.

Reflecting and evaluating – These factors are important because they help both the performers and the observers with their further planning, preparation, adapting and improving. Where standards are satisfactory, there is evidence of:

a recognition of key features and keen and accurate observation

b awareness of accuracy of work

c good self-evaluation and helpful suggestions for improvement

d sensitive concern for another's feelings, and a good choice of words regarding another's work.

Year 5 Dance Programme

Pupils should be able to:

Autumn	Spring	Summer
1 Practise to develop basic skills of travelling, jumping, turning and gesture by linking them together in increasingly complex sequences.	**1** Plan, perform and appraise longer sequences of movement.	**1** Contribute fully to partner and group activity, mixing well and being considerate towards others' ideas.
2 Tackle more complex tasks with enthusiasm and inventiveness.	**2** Recognise the need for physical competence in stillness and in movement.	**2** Express ideas, moods, feelings, and create a simple story in movement, e.g. 'Small Beginnings' as the mountain stream rushes, bubbles, twists and wells into a wide river.
3 Be assisted and encouraged to plan, refine and adapt performance when working alone or with others.	**3** Use winter words on cards as an immediate stimulus to movement, with basic 'Scatter' of the snowflakes being expressed in different ways, using varied qualities, speeds, shapes and tensions.	**3** Learn an international folk dance, e.g. 'Simi Yadech' of Israel, to expand class repertoire, and to inspire almost non-stop, vigorous activity.
4 Show how variety and contrast enhance a performance in a partner's 'Opposites' dance, with changing actions, speeds, effort, shape, direction or level.	**4** Demonstrate versatile, whole-body movement, able to focus on spine, arms, shoulders as well as legs.	**4** Work in a group to plan and create a dance based on 'Feelings'.
5 Use repeating patterns of movement to enable sequences to be remembered with increasing control and accuracy.	**5** Create a traditional-style folk dance using four of seven figures taught in a circle. Co-operate with three other couples to agree the four repeating figures.	**5** With a partner, use voice sounds as an accompaniment to observed movement, and in groups using voice sound as an accompaniment to words describing holiday places, activities or foods.
6 Improve the effect of a performance by including moments of stillness within a pattern.	**6** Learn an English set dance as a contrast to the created circle dance.	**6** Display capacity for vigorous but neat, whole-hearted but poised, thoughtful, well-planned practising and performing.
7 Use action words on cards to inspire actions; with partners commenting for an improvement; and partner's percussion providing the rhythm.	**7** Repeat a series of movements performed previously. A 'Favourite Dance' can be requested.	**7** Be taught to help selves to improve by making simple judgements on performances.
8 Create a simple story, e.g. 'Jaws', expressing ideas through whole-body movement.	**8** Plan imaginatively to contrast a partner's actions. 'Anything you can do, I can do differently!'	
9 Observe and describe the expressive features of a dance.	**9** Explain own couple's contrasts and point out those of other couples.	

Year 5

Lesson Plan 1 • 30 minutes
September

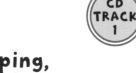

Theme: *Basic actions of travelling, jumping, turning.*

Warm-up Activities
5 minutes

1 Step forwards for three counts and bring feet together on four. Forwards, 2, 3, feet together. Walk backwards for three counts and bring feet together on four. Back, 2, 3, feet together.

2 Again. Forwards, 2, 3, together; back, 2, 3, together; step, 2, 3, feet together; back, 2, 3 and stop!

3 Well done. Now add four sideways stepping movements, starting to the left. It's called a chasse as we step left; close right to left; step left; and close right to left.

4 Now to the right. Step right, close left; step right; close left. To both sides. Left, close; left, close; right close; right, together.

5 Practise your steppings and feet closings to this lively music. Add in a two-beat pause before changes of direction if you want.

Movement Skills Training
15 minutes

1 Can you plan your own pattern? Decide on the number of steps in each direction, with or without pauses.

2 Add in one jump somewhere. Where will it be? At the start or finish? To change direction? Within your stepping? You choose, then keep practising your whole pattern.

3 Now add a spin. Keep the present pattern going. Keep your newly added jump, and somewhere add a spin, small or large.

4 A long, slow spin will be easier to follow. Is your hand, arm or shoulder leading you around into your turn? Make it obvious.

5 Make your stepping, jumping, turning into a repeating, flowing pattern – always in time with the music.

6 Find a partner and show each other your pattern.

Dance — Stepping, Jumping, Spinning, Gesturing
10 minutes

1 With your partner, decide how you will combine your actions so that you are both represented in a steps, jump and spin dance.

2 As you dance together, are you following a leader; facing each other; side by side; or going away from each other and coming back again?

3 Finally, to complete your partners dance sequence, can you add a gesture – of triumph, success, pride, pleasure, or whatever, to make me have a special look at your pair?

4 Your gesture can be anywhere. At the start, it can be a way of gathering for 'Let's go!' At the end it can be a way of saying 'We're brilliant, aren't we!'

5 Pairs, always look for good spaces as you practise, repeat, improve and remember all of your: stepping; jumping; spinning; gesturing (illustrated).

6 Let's have each half of the class looking at and commenting on the other half. Look out for and tell me about the partners and their actions that you particularly liked. I might also ask you to suggest something helpful to make a performance even more admirable.

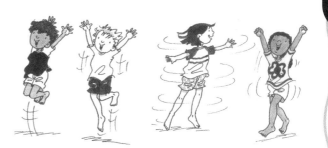

Dance

Teaching notes and NC guidance
Development over 3 lessons

Pupils should be taught to:

a recognise the safety risks of wearing inappropriate clothing, footwear and jewellery
b respond readily to instructions
c be mindful of others.

The setting of standards, an explanation of what is and is not acceptable, should take place during the first lessons of a new school year. This becomes increasingly necessary as pupils become older. This NC requirement is concerned with the way pupils dress, listen, behave, work and show regard for others sharing the space. Badly-dressed classes wear jewellery, for example, watches, rings, necklaces; large, fashionable, un-giving, noisy trainers; long trousers or leg coverings that catch heels; too many layers of clothing; the clothes they wore to school; long hair that is unbunched and impedes vision.

  Badly-behaved classes contain some pupils who talk incessantly; do not listen to or respond to the teacher; need instructions repeated time after time; do not start or stop when told to; disturb and upset others by their selfish, noisy, unsafe rushing around; and work at a pitifully low, half-hearted level, destroying lesson enjoyment for the majority of pupils and the teacher.

  A safe environment requires a well-dressed, well-behaved, quiet, attentive and responsive class. Good behaviour must be pursued continually until it becomes the normal, expected way to work. There is nothing to talk about, apart from those occasions when comments are asked for, usually after a demonstration, or when partners quietly discuss their response to a task.

Warm-up Activities

1–2 The quickest way to teach these steps is for the teacher to stand at the front of the class, so that all are able to see and copy the steps to the lively music. Teacher steps backwards, class step forwards, mirroring one another. 'Your left foot steps forwards, first. Ready? Left, right, left, feet together. Going back, right foot first, now. Right, left, right, feet together.'

3–5 Still facing the class, the teacher now points to what is left for the class. 'Left, close, left, feet together. Back again to your right, now. Right, left, right, feet together.'

Movement Skills Training

1–5 Many will stay with the four-step phrases, and two repetitions of each is ideal. Forwards and back, twice; to left and to right, twice. A jump comes easily at the end of each travel: 'Forwards, 2, 3 and jump,' where on '3' the pupils have stepped on to the left foot then pushed into a jump from the same left foot. After the landing, the right foot starts the travel backwards. 'Back, 2, 3 and jump.' A gentle spin-turn on the spot, turning around with one arm pull, one way, for four counts; and then turning back the other way, other arm leading into the turn, is a good contrast to the livelier steps and jumps. The steppings forwards and back with jumps; stepping side to side with jumps; turnings; all repeated, make a satisfying, flowing pattern.

6 Partners watching each other to plan a combined steps, jumps and spins dance will be thinking particularly of what relationship they will use.

Stepping, Jumping, Spinning, Gesturing Dance

This partners dance, danced to slow, jazzy music, is quickly learned. A gesture of pride or happiness at the end is usual, almost as a reflection on 'our' performance. Pairs can punch the air, together, repeated as in the rest of the dance.

Lesson Plan 2 • 30 minutes
September/October

Theme: *Contrasting actions.*

Warm-up Activities
5 minutes

1 Tiptoe silently, pretending someone is asleep and you must not wake them. Tiny, little, gentle steps. Shhhhh!

2 Pretend the floor is a drum now, and you want your loud, heavy beating to be heard above all the others. Go! Bang! Bang! Bang!

3 Travel with your feet never leaving the floor as you slide, slither and glide along the surface of the floor making very little sound. Slowly, softly, skim along the surface of the floor.

4 Now the floor is red hot and you leap and bound to keep high above it. Bounce and bounce and leap up high.

Movement Skills Training
12 minutes

1 In addition to the gentle and strong, light and heavy contrasts we have practised, we can use fast and slow, and direction change contrasts. Think of a favourite travelling action, using your feet.

2 As I call out 'Normal!' or 'Slow motion!' or 'Fast forwards!' or 'Direction!' can you change the speed or direction of your action? Ready? Normal... fast forwards... slow motion... normal... direction... fast forwards... normal... slow motion... direction... stop!

3 Well done. Your responses were immediate and very contrasting.

4 Can you make a pattern with two pairs of opposites? Aim for variety as well as contrast. For example, can your changes include actions, body shape, direction, speed or force?

5 The medium-speed, rhythmic music is quick enough for stepping and travelling, but slow enough for turns, gestures and big body movements with its 1, 2, 3, 4; opposite, 2, 3, 4 rhythm. Begin.

Dance — Opposites
13 minutes

1 Well done. I saw many good examples of 'Opposites'. Find a partner and take turns at showing each other your four-part sequence with its two pairs of opposites.

2 Partners, can you now plan a four-part sequence, using the best of your two routines, ideally with a good and varied mixture?

3 Keep practising and chant out the nature of your opposites. For example, 'Slow and soft, on the spot; quick and strong, travelling; rise and open, 3, 4; lower and close, 3, 4.'

4 If you prefer, you can repeat each half of your pattern to make your sequence last longer.

5 Finally, decide if you will perform the movements together; or have one do the first movement alone with the other showing the opposite and contrasting movement alone. Working alone can be interesting with one on the spot, the other travelling around the stationary one. In rising and falling, for example, you would be holding opposite shapes at the end.

6 Let's have each half watching the other half to look out for and identify imaginative ideas and neat performances.

7 Thank you for your varied and interesting demonstrations and your friendly, helpful comments. Let's have more practice so that you can include any of the good ideas seen and praised to help improve your performances.

Dance

Teaching notes and NC guidance
Development over 3 lessons

Pupils should be taught to:

a be physically active. Good dress, good behaviour, an instant response to instructions, an unselfish sharing of floor space and consideration for others are the initial priorities to be pursued with a new class. The next priority is to make the lessons physically demanding, with pupils working whole-heartedly and almost non-stop. There is world of difference between a half-hearted, undemanding way of working, and vigorous, energetic, whole-body involvement, using joints and muscles to their maximum potential.

b compose and control their movements by varying shape, size, level, direction, speed and tension. Many times during their Dance lessons, the teacher will have told the class that variety and contrast within a performance enhance and improve the appeal of the performance. An 'Opposites' dance reminds them of examples of variety and contrast within movement.

Pupils should be able to show that they can respond imaginatively to the various challenges. The challenge to 'Plan a four-part sequence with two pairs of "opposites"' is pupil-centred, with ample opportunity to be original, creative and highly imaginative. The challenge for the teacher is to see good examples of such imaginative creativity, and to share it with the class.

Warm-up Activities

1–4 The practising of 'opposites' starts straight away in this lesson. Silent and gentle, and loud, firm feet; light, easy glides and energetic, high leaps and bounces are good examples of contrasting actions and good ways to teach an understanding of what is meant by 'contrast'.

Movement Skills Training

1–5 Speed and direction changes, while travelling, are other obvious examples of contrasts. The teacher's choices of speed change travelling – normal, slow, fast – are to be accompanied by the pupils' own choices of direction changes. Giving praise for immediate responses at the start of a new school year gives the teacher great pleasure. The gentle and strong; light and heavy; fast and slow; forwards and backwards movements, already experienced, are now joined by shape changes (big and small, curled and arched, straight and twisted) contrasts as contributors to variety.

Opposites Dance

1–7 This partners-watching-partners start to the dance climax of the lesson is used often when partners are challenged to 'use the best of your two routines'. In this dance, they are reminded that their decision should be based on aiming for 'a good and varied mixture'. Since each one has two pairs of opposites, ideally they will choose two from each partner's sequence, rather than a three and a one. As they practise the four parts, each dancer can chant his or her pair of opposites as a reminder for both dancers. For example, 'Tap (gently with a foot on the floor, straight arms by the sides) and bounce (firmly with strong arms bending forwards); jump (quickly with feet parting), slide (feet sliding together slowly); forwards (step), sideways (step); out (wide arms reaching) in (arms closing into chest).'

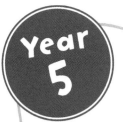

Lesson Plan 3 • 30 minutes
October/November

CD TRACK 7

Theme: *Patterns.*

Warm-up Activities
5 minutes

1 Let's all clap to this folk-dance music and feel its eight-count phrasing. Clap, 2, 3, 4, 5, 6, 7, repeat.

2 Let me clap the first four beats and you do the last four in each phrase. Ready? Me, 2, 3, 4; you, 2, 3, 4; me, 2, 3, 4; you, 2, 3, stop!

3 Now do eight travelling steps, keeping with the music's rhythm. Travel, 2, 3, 4, 5, 6, 7, again. Travel, 2, 3, 4, 5, 6, 7, again.

4 Travel again, but be still on four of the eight beats. Then listen very carefully to the beat to join back in again. It could be 'Still, still, 3, 4; travel, travel, 3, 4', or 'Travel, 2, 3, 4; still, 2, 3, 4'. You decide where your 'action gaps' will be. Begin!

Movement Skills Training
15 minutes

1 Let's try a pattern of eight claps on the spot with little leg action (for example, little bounces in knees); then an eight-count travelling; then clapping on the spot; then travelling.

2 Try an 'action gap' on four of the claps, and four of the travelling steps. Listen carefully, counting to yourself, to join in again.

3 Good. Most of you kept in time, counting through the gaps.

4 On the spot, this time, pretend the floor is a drum as you make rhythmic sounds with your lively feet – bouncing, stamping, jumping, hopping or running. You can clap, also, if you wish.

5 Travel for eight counts in a way that contrasts with your earlier travelling. For example, tiny, long or wide steps; more gentle or more vigorous; fast or slow; sideways or backwards; curving around in a circle instead of straight.

6 Now for our four-part pattern – clapping on the spot with little leg action; travelling; lively feet on the spot; travel to show a contrast with previous travel. Get ready. Begin.

Dance – Partners and patterns
10 minutes

1 Find a partner and show each other your four-part repeating pattern. While you are watching, count to eight to check that your partner is exactly in time with each phrase of the music.

2 Plan to combine two of your own and two of your partner's actions to make your shared pattern. Practise until you can remember and repeat it. Quietly clap, 3, 4, 5, 6, now you travel; travel, 2, 3, 4, 5, 6, now on the spot; lively feet, 3, 4, 5, 6, 7, 8; different travel, different travel, 5, 6, 7, repeat.

3 Well done. I saw lots of interesting variety. Variety also comes from the ways that you work as a pair. You can have one on the spot and one travelling during each phrase of the music. You can face each other on the spot, then travel, side by side; or follow a leader; or part and close. Discuss, decide, practise please.

4 Well done. Can each of you now include one four-count stillness? Where will you do this? At the start, finish or in the middle? Both in the same place or not? Where do you think it will be most dramatic to hold a pause and an interesting body shape?

5 Let's see if you can keep in time with the music, without my counting, as you keep repeating your four-part pattern. We can then have a look at couples still in time with the music at the end.

Dance

Teaching notes and NC guidance
Development over 3 lessons

Pupils should be taught to be mindful of others. The 'others', in this case, include the remainder of the class with whom they are sharing the floor space. It might be necessary to practise travelling 'along straight lines, never following another' as you visit all parts of the room – the ends, sides and corners as well as the middle. Most primary school children will travel anti-clockwise in a big circle, if not taught otherwise. 'Others' also include the partner with whom pupils are combining unselfishly and co-operatively, listening to and acting upon his or her views for the benefit of the partner work.

Pupils should be able to show that they can repeat sequences with increasing control and accuracy. The ability to plan, practise, improve, learn, remember and repeat a sequence of movements is a main target within the NC. Having a repetitive, rhythmic pattern of two, three or four actions is a great aid to remembering and repeating. When the teacher is able to rhythmically accompany the actions, this helps the partners to keep with the music, and acts as a reminder of what is happening and what comes next. 'Clap on the spot, 3, 4, 5, 6, now we travel; travel, travel, off you go, 5, 6, now on the spot; lively, lively, on the spot, 5, 6, travel again; new action, travel, travel, 5, 6, 7, stop!'

Warm-up Activities

1–4 The alternate teacher and class clapping keeps pupils' attention, which is always a good exercise at the start of the lesson. Travelling to the music for groups of eight counts is assisted, at first, by the teacher's chanting. Travelling for four, alternating with being stationary for four, is an excellent challenge, particularly if the teacher does not always call out 'Travel, 2, 3, 4; still 2, 3, 4' to help them.

Movement Skills Training

1–6 This challenging development of a pattern or sequence of linked actions progresses from:

a 8 claps on the spot with a small leg action, alternating with 8 travelling steps; to

b 4 claps and 4 still hands, alternating with 4 travelling steps and 4 still feet; to

c 8 lively, strong foot actions on the spot, alternating with 8 travelling steps that contrast with the 8 travel steps in (a); to

d the eventual, four-part, repeating pattern – clapping on the spot with gentle leg actions; travelling; vigorous feet on the spot, with claps, if wished; travelling with contrasting actions to the earlier travelling – requires thoughtful planning and practising.

Partners and Patterns Dance

1–5 Showing a partner your four-part pattern; watching your partner's pattern; and then planning a four-part sequence to include work from both partners, is often used as a lead-up to partner work, which is one of the most co-operative, friendly and enjoyable experiences in Dance. The order of the sequence, introduced by the teacher, is retained, making the task easier to remember. The changes of relationships as they travel, and the inclusion of moments of four-count stillness, always in time with the music, becomes the lesson's challenging climax.

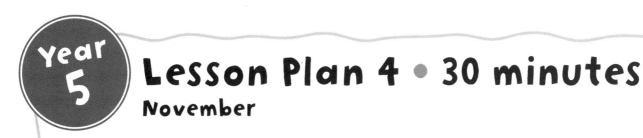

Lesson Plan 4 • 30 minutes
November

Theme: *Action words with percussion accompaniment.*

Warm-up Activities
5 minutes

1 An earlier lesson was about contrasting movements. The way I sound my tambourine will tell you how I want you to move. Can you recognise and respond to slow or quick; quiet or loud; soft or vigorous; big or little; even happy or sad? Ready? Go!

2 Good. I liked your speedy responses to my changing rhythms.

3 Show me your movements to my loud banging alternating with my gentle tapping. Space out well and visit all parts of the room.

4 Now show me your actions to my shaking alternating with my smooth rubbing of the tambourine.

Movement Skills Training
15 minutes

1 All show me a travelling action to my tambourine accompaniment. When I stop playing, be perfectly still. When I re-start, travel again. Listen for my silences! Go!

2 Please find a partner. One of you collect a piece of percussion. The other collect one set of three cards and place them down on the floor in front of you in their numbered order, 1, 2, then 3. Study the words and plan how you will dance the actions.

3 Dancers, stand ready to perform your three actions on your little stage. Partners, watch carefully so that you can make helpful comments. Without percussion at this stage, start when you are ready.

4 Well done, dancers. Now sit down and be given some friendly, helpful advice to improve your performance. Were the actions clear? Were the body shapes full and clear? Was the timing good or was it too rushed, or too long? Partners, tell them what was good, but also tell them how to improve.

5 The same dancers again, please. Partners with percussion, you may quietly accompany your partner, starting and stopping to make the three actions distinct and separate. Begin when ready.

6 Well done, everyone. The improvements were obvious. Let's have one more practice, then we'll change places, dancers and percussionists.

Dance — Pairs with Percussion
10 minutes

1 All hide the words on your cards now and sit beside another couple who do not know what your three actions are. Each couple has a turn at presenting their dance and the watching couple have to try to identify the three actions being performed. Both partners can have a turn as dancer and as percussionist to give the observers a second look.

2 Percussionists, remember to stop and start each action to keep them separate. Play quietly so that you do not disturb other couples. First couples, please begin.

3 Well done, first couples. I am pleased to hear that most of the watchers were able to recognise and name your three actions. Now change places, please, and start again.

4 Well done, second couples, and very observant watchers.

5 Now I will choose some couples. Can you recognise their actions?

Examples of:
Set 1: LEAP, DRIFT, RUSH, SLITHER, DASH, CREEP, DART
Set 2: GROW, STRETCH, TWIST, OPEN, BEND, SOAR, RISE, SWAY
Set 3: FREEZE, MELT, COLLAPSE, FADE, SCATTER, SHRIVEL, CRUMBLE

Dance

Teaching notes and NC guidance
Development over 3 lessons

Pupils should be taught to:

a respond readily to instructions. There are a lot of helpful instructions in the teaching and development of this dance. At each stage, the dancer and the musician must listen carefully as the little dance grows from the teacher-led, with no percussion, to the final, percussion-led version.

b respond to a range of stimuli, through Dance. There is a triple stimulus here. The words provide the movement content; the partner comments, half-way through development, provide a quality stimulus; the percussion provides the rhythm.

Warm-up Activities

1–4 Listening, and responding thoughtfully to varied tambourine soundings, is an excellent exercise in gaining attention at the start of the lesson. It also requires a quality response – 'What speed?' 'How vigorous or gentle?' 'How big and important or small?' – which will become the theme of the lesson. Responding appropriately to varied sounds is an important part of learning to express feelings or ideas through body movements.

Movement Skills Training

1–6 Dancing to action words on a card to tambourine sounds from a partner is taught and developed as follows: (a) dancer performs the three actions, watched very carefully by a partner who does not play the tambourine yet; (b) dancer sits beside observing partner to be told something encouraging and positive, and something that might improve the sequence; (c) dancer, having been coached, repeats the performance, now accompanied by the tambourine; (d) teacher asks tambourine partners to put up their hands if they thought that their partners had improved, asking some observers to explain the improvement; and (e) partners change places to repeat the learning pattern.

Pairs with Percussion Dance

From the teacher's controlling of the timing of the dancing of each of the three words in the middle of the lesson, with 'First action... go! Second action... go! Third action... go!', the next stage is to have all the dancers and tambourinists start on the teacher's 'First action, begin!' and then each tambourinist sounds out the appropriate lengths of sounds to fit the nature of the three actions. Some actions, like 'shoot' are short and quick. Others, like 'drift' are longer because they are slower. Tambourinists need to be told to play quietly and not disturb the groups next to them. They also need to be told to pause, in silence, between sound makings so that the dancer can hold a still body shape that fits the previous action, in between actions, and wait to hear the next sound to respond to. The class at the end can be asked 'Watch Scott and Rebecca who are working really well. Try to recognise and tell me what are the three action words on their turned-over card. Then tell me what was in their actions that impressed you.' Hopefully, the clear actions; firm, clear body shapes; good use of speed; correct use of effort and body tension; and, simply, the whole-hearted, enthusiastic, eye-catching participation will be mentioned.

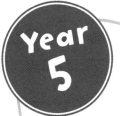

Year 5

Lesson Plan 5 • 30 minutes
December

CD TRACKS 25+29

Theme: *Storytelling.*

Warm-up Activities
5 minutes

1 Pretend you are 'winter-sunning' in the sea on some tropical island – well away from our miserable December weather. Show me two or three swimming actions to this slow music.

2 Walk, showing me your graceful, relaxed swimming strokes. This is the life!

3 Share the 'water space' sensibly, slowly turning arms in front, back or to the side. Weave in and out of each other.

4 If you are swimming backwards, look over one shoulder from time to time.

5 Can you tread water and bob up and down?

6 Make a little repeating pattern. It could be breaststroke; tread water; sink; push up and back stroke. You decide, then practise it.

Movement Skills Training
15 minutes

1 At the start of our 'Jaws' dance, the shark is lurking in the corner of the room, crouched low to the floor, in a long shape with arms reaching along the floor, legs stretched out to the rear. Our two sharks, Sue and Tony, can practise from the same corner to start with.

2 The rest of the class, in the opposite corner, are unaware of the danger. Sharks, look at them, but do not move yet.

3 Sharks, rise slowly. Creep towards the centre of the room, looking at the swimmers.

4 Sharks, swim from side to side at the centre of the room, still a good distance away. Some of you swimmers see the threat and your movements become agitated and quicker.

5 Sharks, move away again towards your starting corner, turn and move right down the room.

6 Sharks, move from side to side, then close in and circle right around the group in the corner, and finish at the front again.

7 Swimmers, you are now anxious, expressing your fear in rapid arm and shoulder gestures, swimming out of the way in panic.

Dance – Jaws
10 minutes

Music: *The Water Kite* sequence from *Jaws* by John Williams (1 min 30 secs)

Group dance with two groups, one at each end of the hall. Each group contains 'Jaws', and several swimmers.

Time	
0 secs	'Jaws', hide low in your corner. Swimmers, enjoy the sea.
20 secs	'Jaws', rise, approach the group, then return almost to your corner.
30 secs	'Jaws', advance half-way to the swimmers. Swimmers, some of you become frightened and start to panic.
40 secs	Sharks, rush from side to side, trapping swimmers in the corner, then circle the swimmers.
1 min 10 secs	Sharks, rush in and grab a swimmer who falls to the floor, trying to resist. 'Jaws', grip your victim, side on by arm and a leg, and drag him or her, slowly, along the floor, away from the other frightened, helpless swimmers reaching both arms towards the victim.
1 min 30 secs	'Jaws', complete the pull on your victim at the room. Swimmers form a close group, low and long stretched, facing and still reaching up and out towards the victim.

Dance

```
          J              SSS
        V                SSS
                         SSS
                          SS
           S              S
         SS
       SSS
     SSS                V
   SSS                J
```

J = Jaws, V = Victims, S = Swimmers

Teaching notes and NC guidance
Development over 3 lessons

Pupils should be able to:

a create simple characters and stories.

b express feelings, moods and ideas. Creating characters and expressing ideas is easier if there is a clearly understood, easily visualised setting in which the characters and expressions are happening. An isolated 'Can you show me how to express fear?' does not conjure up a helpful image that can be translated into something specific.

Pupils should be able to show that they can plan imaginatively, perform to convey ideas, and reflect on the performance and suggest ways to improve it.

Warm-up Activities

1–7 This is the calm, relaxed, carefree swimming before the terror and panic that is coming to the same waters. Most of the water-space actions are dictated by the teacher to provide good variety. Without such teacher-direction, there might only be breaststroke swimming. The mixture of strokes and directions; the treading of water; the sinking to the bottom and the push back up with more swimming; and the repeating five-part pattern all combine to make this an interesting activity and start to the lesson. The 'mood' of the swimmers will be relaxed and happy, without a care in the world.

Movement Skills Training

1–7 With the swimmers and the two sharks in their starting positions, the teacher needs to explain what will happen and then dictate each part of the dance. 'Swimmers, continue the calm, happy, relaxed, varied swimming movements that we have just practised.' 'Sharks, in your corner, stay low and out of sight, looking at, but not moving towards the swimmers.' 'Sharks, slowly creep forwards, but keep low, still out of sight, into the middle of the room.' 'Swimmers, still unaware of trouble, keep swimming, weaving in and out of one another.' 'The nearest group of swimmers see the sharks and react with quicker, distressed movements.' 'Sharks, swim away from the swimmers, as if you are leaving, then come back at them quickly, cornering them.' 'Sharks, zigzag and then circle right around the swimmers, making them feel trapped.' 'Swimmers, whose previous body movements expressed your calm and carefree feelings, change now to rapid body movements expressing anxiety, fear, terror.'

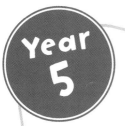

Lesson Plan 6 • 30 minutes
January

CD TRACK 30

Theme: *Winter words and group activity.*

Warm-up Activities
5 minutes

1   This slow, gentle music makes me think of bubbles or balloons flying. Show me how you might choose to move on the spot in response to the music.

2   As you twist and turn, do you feel high, balancing on tiptoes? 'Hovering lightly' might describe your floating movements.

3   Travel now, drifting lightly and slowly from space to space. You have no weight and the air carries you, up and down, around and around, sometimes curving, sometimes on straight lines as you weave in and out of one another, like a snowflake.

Movement Skills Training
15 minutes

1   Join together in groups of five. Make a circle shape and show me your own starting shape as you represent a falling snowflake. Turn on the spot on tiptoes, held in space.

2   Can you travel, in and out of one another, close but not touching as you swirl, hover, float, curving and gliding – like a snowflake in the winter wind?

3   Well done, weightless dancers. Now relax and discuss how your three-part pattern will end. Will you make a frozen shape suddenly?; all drop, gently together?; scatter away to land at different places?; or join together to make a beautiful snowflake shape? When you are ready, practise.

4   Let's try your three-part pattern now. Ready? Lightly on the spot, high and weightless; travel, in and out, floating, twisting and turning. Now your own finish, please.

5   Very well done, with many attractive finishes. Let's look at two groups at a time and comment on the ideas and actions that we liked, and any impressions of good 'group togetherness'.

Dance — Winter Words and Group Actions
10 minutes

1   Stay in your groups of five and I will give each group a card. Every card has the word 'Scatter' on it, but there are four different versions of how snowflakes scatter for you to plan and perform as a group. Please do not look at another group's card. Later on, you will be guessing what their words are.

2   Continue practising and I will come around and help you to make your movements clearer. Show me your group's clear, still start and finish positions and shapes. Make your actions neat and try to show the particular movement qualities on your card.

SCATTER/SLOWLY/WITH SAME ACTION VARIED SHAPES ENDING

SCATTER/SWIRLING/ONE AFTER THE OTHER TO SETTLE

SCATTER/DRIFTING/WITH CHANGES OF SPEED TO RE-FORM

SCATTER/FLUTTERING/LIGHTLY SINKING/FREEZING

3   Practise your four-part pattern further. Then we will look at each group in turn to make friendly, helpful comments.

Dance

Teaching notes and NC guidance
Development over 3 lessons

Pupils should be taught to:

a adopt the best possible posture and use of the body. Often in Dance, the focus is on the travelling actions used to transport us. This is particularly true in folk dance, for example. For variety and to promote well-controlled, poised and versatile whole-body movement, we sometimes focus on movements involving the spine, arms and shoulders as well as the legs, as we bend, stretch, twist, turn, curl or arch, expressing movement qualities such as lightness, changing shapes or speed, gentle falling, or a hardening of body tension;

b compose and control their movements by varying shape, size, level, direction, speed or tension. After the question 'What action?', we develop by asking 'What shape?' 'Where is the action happening?' and 'How is the action being performed?' to allow consideration for shape, size, level, direction, speed or tension.

Pupils should be able to show that they can use simple judgements to improve the accuracy, quality and variety of their own performances. Within the dual emphasis on performing and learning which is the basis of NC Physical Education, reflection and evaluation by pupils helps them to adapt, change and plan again, guided by their own and others' judgements.

Warm-up Activities

1–3 The use of imagery stimulates the imagination and helps pupils understand more easily and clearly what is wanted from them. Moving like a balloon or a bubble inspires an immediate and appropriate response. Being simply asked by the teacher to 'Show me how you can move lightly, floating' does not produce the same understanding of the movement qualities involved. The 'hovering, drifting, light movements' can be made even more clear if pupils watch the movements of bubbles being blown by the teacher or pupils. The weightless flying like bubbles, balloons or snowflakes emphasises the 'How?' factor in movement.

Movement Skills Training

1–5 The weightlessness, experienced individually, is now progressed into groups of five who practise, experiment, discuss and agree a pattern of floating lightly on the spot; travelling; and ending their sequence in their own chosen way. While much of Physical Education teaching involves vigour and lively actions to stimulate much-needed, challenging activity, this lesson concentrates on the contrasting, gentler, softer movement qualities, because the inclusion of such contrasting elements within movement makes a huge contribution to the attractiveness of performances.

Winter Words and Group Actions Dance

1–3 The same groups of five stay together and are challenged to co-operate to plan how to perform as scattering snowflakes in the manner listed on their own card, which is different from that on all the other cards. They will need to agree actions; use of clear body shapes; own and group space, including directions used; changes of speed as they travel; and how to finish, trying to make these elements clear for the eventual demonstrations and comments.

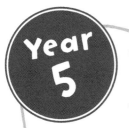

Lesson Plan 7 • 30 minutes
January/February

CD TRACK 20

Theme: *Traditional, folk-dance style, creative dance.*

Warm-up Activities
5 minutes

1   Skip freely by yourself, to visit all parts of the room.

2   Travel along straight lines, not curving around, following others.

3   When drum sounds twice, join with the nearest person and dance.

4   When drum sounds once, separate and dance by yourself.

5   When drum sounds twice, find a different partner from the one you had last time.

Figures that can be used in a Circle Formation
15 minutes

Each figure takes eight counts of the music. Partners are all in one big circle where they can see the teacher and do easily supervised practice together. A boy dances on the left of the pair.

1   All walk into the centre and out again.

2   Boys alone skip into the centre, then out again.

3   Girls dance into the centre and out again.

4   Chasse with partner, hands joined, into the centre and out again. (Step sideways to centre with nearer foot; close other foot to first foot; step sideways to centre; close other foot. Side, close; side, close; 3 and 4. Step out, close; out, close; 3; and 4.)

5   Join hands in a circle and slip to left and back to right.

6   Perform a Grand Chain, giving alternate hands to the person coming towards you. (Boys travel anti-clockwise, all giving right hands to the first person met.)

7   Promenade, side by side, nearer hands joined, anti-clockwise around in a big circle.

Circles of Four Couples Plan and Practise Own Dance
10 minutes

1   Each couple chooses to include one of the seven figures above. Try to make your dance interesting with variety and contrast – all dancing, then only a few; movements into the circle and out, as well as around in a circle; movements forwards and/or backwards and/or sideways, for example. Each make your choice and practise.

2   Remember there are eight counts to each figure in your four-figure folk dance. Get into the habit of counting in groups of eight.

3   Let us look at each circle in turn. Please look out for and tell me which circle linked its actions smoothly together and included interesting variety and contrast.

4   Thank you, performers and those making helpful comments. Before we continue practising for improvement, can you think of any features of folk dance that improve its appearance?

5   Yes, circles that stay round; neat footwork, always in time with the music, never late or early; good teamwork and being ready to come in at the right time and place; and a general impression of enthusiasm and enjoyment.

Dance

Teaching notes and NC guidance
Development over 3 lessons

Pupils should be taught to:

a be physically active. One of the best ways to ensure that pupils are almost non-stop physically active is through folk dance lessons. The music provides the continuous accompaniment; the steps and figures are lively; and for most of the dances, all couples in the circle are dancing.

b be mindful of others. Being 'mindful of others' means sensibly and unselfishly sharing space when practising, and co-operating considerately in agreeing and planning the four-figure repeating pattern of the created dance.

c perform a number of dances from different times and places, including some traditional dances of the British Isles. The seven figures taught are typical patterns from English and Scottish country dance. The music is traditional. The emphasis on partners working together, thoughtfully and carefully as part of a larger team, is typical of traditional dance.

d repeat sequences with increasing control and accuracy. The repeating pattern of four figures is helped by the teacher counting out the eight-bar phrases of the music for each part, and by the whole class thinking ahead and remembering what comes next. Increasing accuracy depends on the teacher asking for one element to be focused on, and improved, each time.

Warm-up Activities

1–5 This easy, instant, warm-up activity keeps pupils' attention as they listen for the next drum beat telling them to change from dancing alone, to joining a partner, to dancing alone. Such attention-inducing activities are always a good way to start.

Figures that can be used in a Circle Formation

1 With nearer hands joined, partners walk into centre, facing forwards, and walk out to circle, travelling backwards.

2–3 In the skipping into the centre, boys alone, girls alone, once again they face forwards, going in to centre, and come out backwards to places in circle.

4 Partners face each other, with hands joined, to chasse sideways into and out of circle. In a chasse we step to one side, close other foot, step, close.

5 The quick slip-step sideways in the circle is like a skipping chasse step sideways for eight counts. Because it is so lively, dancers need to stop travelling sideways on count six, bring their feet together and under control on counts 7 and 8, ready to travel, slip-stepping back, anti-clockwise to starting places in the circle. 'Slip left, 2, 3, 4, 5, 6, feet together; slip right, 2, 3, 4, 5, 6, feet together.'

6 Turn right hand and shoulder towards the first dancer you meet as you start to progress around the Grand Chain, giving right hand and left hand alternately. Each giving of hands takes one count of the music.

7 The promenade, anti-clockwise around the circle, side by side with partner, is easy. The teacher's reminder here is to 'Keep your nice big circle round, please!'

Circles of Four Couples Plan and Practise Own Dance

One dancer from each of the four pairs can say the actions of the figure chosen by that pair, as a reminder. Ideally, the final figure will be one involving all eight dancers in the set, non-stop.

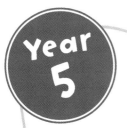
Lesson Plan 8 • 30 minutes
February/March

CD TRACKS 9 + 10

Theme: *Traditional folk dance.*

Warm-up Activities
5 minutes

Partners in a big circle, all face anti-clockwise, right hands joined, boys on the inside.

1   Do eight skipping steps forwards, side by side, in the circle.

2   Face your partner and, without contact, do four setting steps. (Step to side; close other foot to first foot; mark time on the spot with first foot. Step, close, beat. To side, close, beat. Later a jump is added to the first step. Jump, 2, 3; jump, mark time; side, 2, 3.)

3   Change places with partner, giving right hands for four counts.

4   Face partner and do four setting steps. (Right, 2, 3; left, 2, 3; right, 2, 3; left, 2, 3.)

5   Change back to own places, giving left hands for four counts.

6   Eight skipping steps around, side by side, right hands joined, anti-clockwise in the circle.

Keep repeating.

Teach and Dance – Three Meet (English Folk Dance)
18 minutes

Music: *Three Meet* by Blue Mountain Band or any 32 bar reel tune.

The grand circle around the room is made of trios facing trios. A boy with a partner on each hand faces a girl with a partner on each hand.

Bars 1–8   Trios, advance to meet and retire. Then, still facing the other trio, change places, dropping hands to pass one another.

Bars 9–16   Repeat the advancing and retiring, and the passing to change places, back to original places (illustrated).

Bars 17–24   All six join hands in a ring and circle to the left, then change direction and circle back, right, to places.

Bars 25–32   Each trio should form a ring, circle left and as the two rings circle, pass each other by revolving around each other and so progress on one place in the grand circle.

Each line of three dancers now opens up to face a new trio to repeat the dance.

Revise a Favourite Dance
7 minutes

This can be a folk dance such as 'Cumberland Reel', 'Djatchko Kolo', 'Farmer's Jig' or 'Wrona Gapa' from previous lessons, or, for variety, a creative dance learned and remembered earlier in the school year. Such a dance, using more modern music or no music, and involving the class in movements different from the traditional steps and patterns above, will produce the interesting and varied content that makes a lesson satisfying for everyone.

Dance

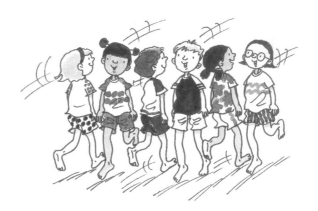

Teaching notes and NC guidance
Development over 3 lessons

Pupils should be taught to:

a be physically active and engage in activities that develop the heart and lungs. Near non-stop action is a general feature of folk dance lessons. Continuous use of the big leg muscles inspires healthy development of the heart and lungs – body parts, according to the experts, seldom used for prolonged periods by modern, mostly sedentary youngsters.

b perform a number of dances from different times and places, including some traditional dances of the British Isles. 'Three Meet' is a popular English folk dance, often included to give interesting variety to a dance programme. Unusually, it is made up of trios facing trios in a big circle, all around the room. It is, equally unusually, a progressive dance with all trios, facing anti-clockwise or clockwise, moving on one place in that direction after each completion of the dance, to meet and dance with a new trio.

Pupils should be able to show that they can repeat a series of movements performed previously. By now, the extensive class repertoire should mean that the teacher will receive an encouraging response to the question 'Which favourite dance shall we end the lesson with?' One of the many attractions of folk dances is that they have a long 'shelf life' and pupils are happy to repeat them.

Warm-up Activities

1–6 This warm-up, with its skipping in and out of the circle; setting to partners; changing places with partners; setting to partners; and skipping around in the circle, is like a complete little dance. It is easy apart from the setting steps to partners which need to be introduced, demonstrated and taught. For complete beginners, a flat-footed left, right, left; right, left, right on the spot with the music will suffice.

Teach And Dance – Three Meet

With the trios facing trios, all around the room, ready to start, the teacher says 'Hands up the trios who are facing this way (anti-clockwise); the other way (clockwise). Good. Please remember that you will always be facing this way in this dance. Look ahead to the two trios next to you in our big class circle. Point to the three in that group who are facing you. That group of three in the next circle will be the trio you meet and dance with after one completion of the dance.'

Revise a Favourite Dance

With a class who are exceptionally keen on Dance, a list of their dance repertoire on a classroom notice board will remind them of dances they have particularly liked and remembered. Before coming to the hall, they can decide which dance to include at the end, 'if you work hard, as usual, and learn the new folk dance.' By knowing beforehand, the teacher can be sure to have the correct music, if music is needed.

Lesson Plan 9 • 30 minutes
March

Theme: *Contrasts in movement.*

Warm-up Activities
5 minutes

1 Showing 'contrasts' in our movements means showing clearly how they are different. One obvious contrast is travelling and being still. Please show me an example, from a still starting position.

2 Good. Same again, but with this half of the room showing soft, gentle travelling into a slow, graceful stop, while the other half vigorously, firmly travel into a sudden, rigid stop. Go!

3 Very good and very contrasting. This time, the silent, graceful half will move slowly through only a short distance travel and finish in a small, 'easy' body shape. The vigorous, lively half will travel far and finish in a wide, firm body shape. Go!

Movement Skills Training
10 minutes

1 Find a partner and we'll play at 'Anything you can do, we can do differently!' Partner A, on the spot, show an action your hands can do. Partner B, join in with an action that demonstrates a contrast. It might be clapping, then fingers bending and stretching. Hands only... go! Keep repeating.

2 Well done, partners B. Now you go first, using feet only, on the spot, challenging your partner to do one that contrasts. For example, lightly peeling feet up from floor and loudly stamping feet down on to floor. Feet only... go! Keep repeating.

3 I saw lots of good contrasts. Partners A, can you show B a whole-body movement, on the spot, for them to contrast with?

4 Let's look at some excellent contrasts: rise, fall; open, close; stretch, curl; shake loosely, turn stiffly; and flop, freeze.

Dance — Anything You Can Do, We Can Do Differently!
15 minutes

1 Stay with your partner and find a couple to work with. Couple A will plan travelling actions to a still finish. Couple B will plan whole-body movements on the spot.

2 With your own partner, discuss, plan and practise your actions or movements to show to the other couple.

3 Find a good starting place, pairs of couples, for A to show their travelling actions, then be still. Bs watch, discuss, then follow with contrasting travelling actions. Keep practising your actions, which can include contrasting, still starting and finishing shapes.

4 Excellent. Your groups of four are now working and contrasting well together.

5 B couples, show the other couples your big body movements on the spot. Decide how often you will repeat them before becoming still to wait for the As to discuss and decide how they will contrast with you.

6 Well done, with lots of contrasting actions, shapes, levels and groupings. Now, show me your group starting positions for your whole pattern of contrasting travelling and actions on the spot. Keep going. Go!

7 While each half of the class perform for the other half, those watching, please look out for good examples of contrasts and be able to describe the differences, so that we can all learn.

Dance

Teaching notes and NC guidance
Development over 3 lessons

Pupils should be taught to compose and control their movements by varying shape, size, level, direction, speed and tension. It has been said that every Dance lesson should include contrast and variety, almost like a good meal. The movement elements providing contrast and variety include: changes of shape and size (for example, curled in on oneself, clicking fingers, or huge, explosive, star-shaped leap with full arm extension); changes of level or direction (for example, rising, advancing to high on tiptoes, or sinking and turning on the spot); changes of speed and tension (for example, gently, slowly, gliding and turning, or rushing, reaching, vigorously straight ahead).

Pupils should be able to show that they can respond imaginatively to the various challenges. The pupils plan their own actions in one half of the dance and then plan contrasting actions in the other half. In pupil-centred lessons such as this, with pupils free to be original and creative, the teacher must be observant and demonstrate with good examples so that he or she, and the class, see, enjoy and learn from the good ideas.

Warm-up Activities

1–3 Examples of contrasts here include: on the spot and travelling; easy, gentle travelling with a smooth, relaxed stop and dynamic, strong travelling with a tight stop; graceful short distance travelling and a quiet, calm, small body shape, and exuberant travelling with a huge, strong body shape finish. All the time, the class are focused on examples of contrasts or opposites in dance movement because these contrasts are attention-catchers and often a complete surprise to observers.

Movement Skills Training

1–3 Partners face each other on the spot to practise at a speed suggested by the teacher or one that can be led by a medium speed, jazzy piece of music. 'One (leader moves)... and... two (partner does an opposite action)'; or 'I go... you follow'; or 'My hands... your hands'; or 'My gentle feet... your noisy feet.' Sensible leading partners can quietly say the contrasting actions as an accompaniment and reminder.

Anything You Can Do, We Can Do Differently! Dance

1–7 Partners join up with another couple to work towards a dance made up of two pairs of opposites. Couple A will be responsible for planning travelling actions and couple B have to plan their own, opposite travelling actions. Couple B are responsible for planning big body movements on the spot. Couple A have to plan contrasting on-the-spot actions. Couples watch each other's demonstrations; discuss their ideas for contrasting actions; plan and practise their movements. It becomes a 'Couple A travels; couple B travels; couple B moves on-the-spot; couple A moves on-the-spot' four-part repeating pattern of opposites. For the half-watching-half demonstrations, the teacher asks 'Please look out for and tell me about excellent examples of opposites that you see. Can you see good action, body shape, level, direction, speed or force opposites to tell me about, please?'

Lesson Plan 10 • 30 minutes
April/May

CD TRACK 32

Theme: *Responding to music to express ideas.*

Warm-up Activities
5 minutes

1 In a previous lesson I told you that the piece of music made me think of flying bubbles, balloons or snowflakes. Today's piece of classical music makes me think of the tiny beginnings of a stream from its slow trickling, hillside start, through its rushing, splashing middle over rocks and waterfalls, to its full width, majestic river climax as it travels on towards the sea.

2 Kneel down and let your gentle hand and arm actions make the early trickling, seeping, creeping action of the drops of hill water as they first appear.

3 Rise up higher on your knees to make these curving water patterns become bigger. The curving movements can run out forwards, or they can be a sidewards impression of the tiny water flow, curving out of the hillside, and starting to trickle downwards.

4 Once again, crouch very low. Show me your two first stages, your 'small beginnings' from seeping, small action start to hillside trickle, as you become taller, making the curving actions bigger.

Movement Skills Training
12 minutes

1 On your feet now, show me tiny floor patterns, little curves, on a figure 8 as the new stream drops down a little step, and then swirls back on itself.

2 We did 'contrasts' in our last lesson. Can you contrast these slow curling movements, curling around a bend, with the quicker bubbling over stones?

3 Using hands in space, trace the pattern of the water. Everything so far has been in a small space. We can alternate the gentle, slow, trickling, curving in and out and around on its figure 8, with the bubbling and speeding up

over the small rocks, using hand patterns in space.

4 Make your curving, travelling floor pattern bigger and feel it with your whole body, not just your feet and arms.

5 Your growing stream meanders, curving, swirling, dropping and bubbling over stones and rocks with a rush and a crash.

6 At the waterfalls, change levels, splashing up, then spreading and diving down.

7 Emphasise the interesting contrasts – dashing over rocks; splashing up and spreading and tumbling down; and the long, slow, smoother curving patterns.

8 Still by yourself, use the whole floor space with your big, slow, sweeping curves that change speed as you go around a boulder, along a fast, narrow bit, or crash over a waterfall.

Dance – From Small Beginnings
13 minutes

1 Make groups of three, taking turns to be the leader, who can be crouched like a rock for the other two to negotiate, going over or around. They can follow the leader, speeding through narrows, tumbling down and swirling back on themselves, and crashing out in space before tumbling down the waterfalls.

2 The small tributaries of trios gradually come in from the sides or the centre of the room and join the ever-growing, expanding and widening river, as it settles down to a smoother, steadier, almost uninterrupted flow.

3 Let's try the whole dance from the hillside beginnings and source of it all.

continued overleaf...

Dance

Music: Smetana's *Ma vlast* (My Fatherland), Second Movement, by the Boston Symphony Orchestra (3 mins 44 secs).

Time

0 secs	All start, well-spaced apart, crouched low to the floor. The water seeps out gently and slowly. The rising and sinking of your chest, only, can express 'Something is coming'.
12 secs	Add in gentle arm actions as the river's life starts to appear, with flexible curving patterns by hands only, then arms, then body, still low on the spot.
25 secs	Gradually rise up on to your knees and make your curving patterns bigger. Are you showing the water trickling away ahead of you, down the hill, or from a side-on view?
45 secs	Turn, sometimes in a figure 8, as your stream drops and then turns back on itself. Can you show me both slow, curving movements, around bends in the stream, and faster bubbling as you crash over stones?
1 m	Show me, with your arm movements in space, how your stream expands from its slow, curving and trickling back on itself to its speeding and bubbling over stones.
1 m 25 secs	Use more space as you use your whole body and show the growing line of your expanding stream as it makes its swirling, meandering progress.
1 m 40 secs	Waterfalls, now, and changing levels, as you splash and spread upwards, then dive down to re-join the stream.
1 m 55 secs	By yourself still, use lots of space for your big, slow, sweeping curves that suddenly change speed as you meet a fast, narrow section, or a big boulder, or a sudden waterfall.
2 m 20 secs	In groups of three, take turns at being the leader, sometimes being still for the others to go over or around, and sometimes being the leader, speeding down a narrow section or crashing out in space before you tumble down a waterfall.
2 m 50 secs	Groups of threes come in to join together and make an ever-growing, ever-widening river which settles down, smoothly and steadily, into an almost regular, undisturbed flow.

Teaching notes and NC guidance Development over 4 lessons

Pupils should be taught to:

a respond to music.

b express ideas. Pupils will be asked 'Does the music make you imagine anything? What kind of movements can you see?' When 'Stream or river in the countryside' has been agreed, they can be challenged to suggest ideas for the kinds of movement inspired by the changing phrases of the music – small, slow, on the spot; small, gentle, trickling along; bigger, swirling, using more space; faster, crashing, splashing; stronger, bigger, wider; smoothly, steadily, settling to a quieter, straighter flow.

Warm-up Activities

1–4 The class will need to be informed that the source of a river is often a tiny trickle from quite high up on a hillside. From almost individual droplets at the start, the emerging little stream becomes bigger, more flowing and wider. A trickle has become a flow.

Movement Skills Training

1–8 In this 'shared choice teaching' middle part of the lesson, the teacher decides the order of the dance's content and the stream's progress, and the class decide the exact nature of the actions within each part of the dance.

From Small Beginnings Dance

1 Trios are challenged to work together to express the progress of the expanding stream and the different actions of what will be the rushing, swirling, speeding up and crashing down waterfalls, middle of dance.

2 Groups of small tributaries have progressed their erratic way down the hillside and start to come together as an ever-growing, widening, smoother river progressing towards the sea.

3 With the teacher's continuous reminder of the parts of the dance, and the nature of their actions, the class revises the whole dance from the 'Small Beginnings' start of everything.

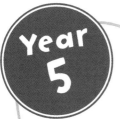

Year 5

Lesson Plan 11 • 30 minutes
May

CD TRACKS 16+19

Theme: *Traditional folk dance.*

Warm-up Activities
6 minutes

1 In your lines of four behind a leader, travel to all parts of the room, looking for good spaces. Focus on and copy your leader's travelling actions. Learn and remember these actions.

2 When I call 'Change!' the leader peels off to the end of the line. Number two leader focuses on the upper body, handclaps and gestures to accompany the known actions.

3 Number three leader concentrates on the size of the steps and the effort being used, contrasting, for example, neat, small, quiet skipping with big, strong, lively, skipping.

4 The last leader concentrates on the 'Where?' and occasionally dances on the spot, alternating with travelling in various directions, not always forwards.

Teach and Dance — Simi Yadech (Israeli Folk Dance)
16 minutes

Music: *Simi Yadech*

A lively dance, performed either in a circle or an open circle with a leader at each end. Start clockwise. Hands are held low.

1 Eight Mayim steps clockwise, starting with right foot, travelling sideways to your left.

2 Travel anti-clockwise, forwards, hands by your sides (illustrated).

  Beat 1 Step forwards on right foot.
  2 Hop on right foot.
  3 Step forwards on left foot.
  4 Hop on left foot.
  5 Step forwards on right foot.
  6 Hop on right foot.

3 As 2 (6 step-hops in all).

4 With body bending forwards quickly, step forwards on right foot; step forwards on left foot; step forwards on right foot; step forwards on left foot.

5 Repeat 4.

Mayim Step:

Beat 1 Step right foot across in front of left foot.
2 Step left foot to left.
3 Step right foot behind left foot.
4 Step left foot to left.

Revise a Favourite Dance or Dances
8 minutes

These can be folk dances such as 'Cumberland Reel', 'Djatchko Kolo', 'Farmer's Jig', 'Wrona Gapa' or 'Three Meet' from previous lessons and years, or, for variety, creative dances learned and remembered.

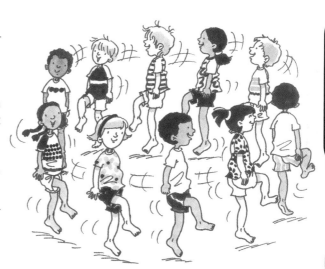

Dance

Teaching notes and NC guidance
Development over 3 lessons

Pupils should be taught to:

a respond readily to instructions. In a quick dance with quite difficult steps, it is essential that all look at and listen to the teacher demonstrating and explaining the actions and the figures of the dance.

b be physically active, engaging in activities that develop the heart and lungs. Folk dances are the most physically demanding areas of a Dance programme. Each lasts for about three minutes of non-stop action, often, as here, with everyone dancing continuously from start to finish. Vigorous action in the big muscles of the legs stimulates and develops the heart and lungs.

c perform a number of dances from different times and places. Certain folk dances, such as this, express the particular style and music of the country's national dance.

Pupils should be able to show that they can repeat and remember a series of movements performed previously. In a folk dance lesson with a well-behaved, responsive class, there should be time at the end of the lesson for the teacher to ask 'Which of your favourite dances would you like to finish with?' or for the teacher to include a dance that he or she would like to revise, or a more gentle dance to contrast with this lively new one.

Warm-up Activities

1–4 Within this 'Follow the Leader', lines of four warm-up, the original leader's sequence of two or three repeating travelling actions has to be repeated and remembered because each new leader will repeat them and enhance them through his or her particular focus. The feet and legs, and the actions they are doing, will be the focus to start with. Two neat travelling actions, particularly if they include a contrast (for example, gentle, tiptoe stepping and lively skipping with high arms and thighs lifting) will be sufficient. Number two leader's focus is on using the upper body to make a clear, firm shape so that they all work harder. Strong, wide or high arm shapes, hand-claps or gestures give the actions greater appeal and interest. Number three leader's focus is on the contrasting sizes and uses of effort that can be applied with the gentle, restrained, and the strong, exuberant contrasts always providing interesting, attractive, eye-catching performances. Since 'Follow the Leader' tends always to be travelling forwards, a focus for leader four, on the 'Where?', will provide ways of using the hall space and the team's movements that the class might not have thought about.

Teach And Dance – Simi Yadech (Israeli Folk Dance)

1 The eight Mayim steps are demonstrated in slow motion by the teacher, standing inside the circle where pupils can all see him or her. 'Look at my feet. The right foot alternates going across in front of, and then going behind, my left foot. My right foot always steps to the left. When I say "In front and behind; in front and behind; in front and behind", I am referring to my right foot movements. On the "and", I step to the left with my left foot.'

2 The six step-hops to the right followed by the quick step, 2, 3, 4 is repeated, still to the right.

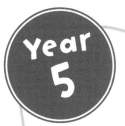

Lesson Plan 12 • 30 minutes
June

Theme: *Feelings.*

Warm-up Activities
5 minutes

1 Skip to this lively folk-dance music with its obvious eight-count phrasing. Keep to the rhythm and feel the sets of eight counts. Go! Skip, 2, 3, 4, 5, 6, 7, 8; travel, travel, 3, 4, find spaces, 7, 8; quietly, neatly, 3, 4, skip and skip, 7, 8; silent skipping, 3, 4, 5, 6, 7, stop!

2 Well done. You all kept exactly with the music. Can you now show me a change with each new group of eight counts? It can be a change of direction, size of steps, body shape within your skipping, or a change of action. Travelling and thinking... begin!

Movement Skills Training
10 minutes

1 Dance lessons, where we express feelings through movement, are difficult. However, you are a brilliant class, so it should be no problem. Show me your proud walking, your proud head and your straight back after being called 'brilliant'.

2 I can see lots of cocky head positions with huge shoulder swaggering. Well done, proud dancers.

3 I am terribly sorry. I made a mistake. You really are a rotten class. Show me your angry stamping, clenching of fists and other movements that express your anger towards me!

4 How dare you stamp your feet at me! You will all be reported and severely punished! Show me a shape that expresses fear. Now travel, showing fear towards something as you creep away, hiding, avoiding, cringing, escaping.

5 Stop creeping away like 'wimps'! Stand up for yourselves! Turn, advance and be aggressive towards the thing or the person. Flex your muscles and get after it. Show who is the boss.

Dance — Feelings
15 minutes

1 Well done, my expressive class. Make groups of five, please.

2 You are going to agree on a feeling that your group would like to express in movement. Ideas on this card include happy; sad; frightened; angry; surprised; aggressive; miserable; exhausted; shy; disgusted; shocked; lonely; bored; puzzled; determined.

3 In your planning, you might want to have one of the group as the focus of your sadness, anger, aggression, shock, fear, misery or whatever. Remember, as you focus with your eyes, it is your body movement that is telling me about your inner feelings.

4 Decide on the size of your little stage; how and where will you move from a still starting position and group shape, through your movement, to your still group positon and shape at the end? You will be able to remember your movements more easily if you have a repeating pattern. (For example, cocky head lift; cocky head lift; swagger, swagger, swagger; or angry stamp, stamp, stamp of feet; punch, punch, punch hand against hand.)

5 Have another two complete practices, then you will present your 'Feelings' dance to the other groups who will be challenged to 'Guess what feelings are being expressed through movement. Can you work out what the focus of these feelings are? (For example, sadness for a dead pet budgie; fear of a monster; aggression towards a bully; disgust towards a litter lout; shocked by an electric current.)'

Dance

Teaching notes and NC guidance
Development over 4 lessons

Physical Education should involve pupils in the continuous process of planning, performing and evaluating. The greatest emphasis should be on the actual performance. In the middle part of the lesson there is a rapid series of challenges to plan and perform a response. 'Show me your proud walking... angry stamping...frightened creeping... aggressive advancing...' There will be several repetitions for improvement, helped by one's own reflecting in response to the teacher's questioning: 'What are the main body movement expressions of pride... anger... fear... aggression?' Reflection guides further planning for an improved performance in this dual physical and educational process. In the group dance climax of the lesson, evaluation will be done by another group who are asked 'Please watch the group and tell me which feelings they are expressing. What movement ideas were particularly clear and expressive? Is there any way they might improve their little dance?

Pupils should be taught to:

a express feelings, moods and ideas.

b respond to a range of stimuli, through Dance. Varied stimuli contribute greatly to pupils' looking forward to Dance lessons. It is hoped, for example, that a range of stimuli (which this year includes actions, percussion, a film story, winter words, traditional folk dances, contrasts, a river, feelings and voice sounds) will provide something of interest for everyone, and help to give the class a varied and interesting repertoire.

Warm-up Activities

1 The teacher can clap or count out the eight-count phrasing of the folk dance music, which is at a good speed for their skipping, finding spaces and visiting all parts of the room.

2 The teacher's 'Ready, change!' on counts 7 and 8 keeps the class together as they try to show some form of change in their travelling and body movements. New travel actions; a different direction; a new, whole, body shape; or smaller, neater or larger, lively steps, changes of effort should all be included or encouraged in this 'thinking warm-up'.

Movement Skills Training

1–5 As the class respond to the teacher's praise, insults, warnings, humiliation, they express the appropriate feelings through their body movements. Because they are imagining themselves in a real situation, the pupils are more easily able to express themselves. Reacting angrily to someone who calls you a 'wimp' is easier than being asked to 'Show me how you might express aggressiveness.' Being told that you are a brilliant class inspires the expression of pride through the body movements of head-held-high swaggering. Other feelings that are easy to express through body actions are happiness, sadness, surprise and weariness.

Feelings Dance

Reference to words on a card provides the groups of five dancers with ideas for their expressed feelings dance. One person as the focus for their feelings is helpful and the class is encouraged to work towards a three- or four-part repeating pattern of body movements, ideally the outcome of their shared group planning of ideas.

Lesson Plan 13 • 30 minutes
July

Theme: *Vocal sounds accompaniment and stimulus for movement.*

Warm-up Activities
5 minutes

1 We can accompany dance with recorded music, instruments, body-part sounds such as clapping, and voice sounds. Follow me as I travel all around the room and accompany me with your good voice sounds, copying my actions. A helpful rhythm will be appreciated.

2 I liked the 'Toom, toom, toom, toom' with my marching; the 'Tick, tock, tick, tock' with my slow, feet-astride stepping; the loud humming as I turned; and the 'Boomp, boomp, boomp, boomp' with my bouncing.

Movement Skills Training
10 minutes

1 Find a partner and decide who is the mover and who is the voice accompaniment. Mover, can you vary your actions, staying on the spot only? Do small, smooth movements for a small, smooth, continuous sound from your partner.

2 Now try a bigger action which might be a stop/start to invite a louder, jerky, on/off sound.

3 Rise and fall, mover, to give your partner an interesting variety of sounds to make. Changing speed would be good to see and hear.

4 Change places, please. The new mover will travel, not too far or fast, with the sound-making partner travelling and making some brilliant, unique sounds.

5 Travelling partner, please vary your actions to include, for example, slow, smooth, jerky, big, small to give your sound-making partner plenty of variety, making sounds never heard before.

6 Let's have each half of the class performing and making sound for the other half. Watch and listen for brilliant partnerships to tell me about, so that we can share really good ideas.

Dance — Voice Sounds
15 minutes

1 Form groups of five. Sit down and discuss a favourite idea for a holidays 'Voice Sounds' dance. You may elongate or shorten action words, (Pl-a-a-a-ay te-e-n-n-is); place names, (The R—i-v-i-i—era); favourite food, (Ba-a-aa-nan-a split); or invent sounds or words to accompany your holiday actions.

2 Are you thinking of an enjoyable holiday sporting action; a favourite holiday resort; or food, glorious food? Start to work out your accompanying actions as a group.

3 Sporting action will be represented by the actions, ultra-slow, normal speed or speeded up, if you can shorten the word.

4 Place names and food can be accompanied by an interesting mixture of travelling, jumping, turning, rising, falling, gesturing and stillness – long, drawn out, normal speed or accelerated to make it eye-catching and funny.

5 Agree your starting shapes and finishing shapes as a group.

6 Try to include actions that make a short repeating pattern to help you to remember them easily. Keep practising.

7 For your demonstrations, one group at a time, try to be expressing 'Our choice of sport, or resort, or food, is the best – just like our movement. Watch how well we work together. Watch our larger-than-life movements and listen to our super sounds.'

Dance

Teaching notes and NC guidance
Development over 3 lessons

Pupils should be able to show that they can:

a respond imaginatively to the various challenges. Both partners are being challenged to make imaginative and very different responses. 'Mover, can you...? Sound accompanist, can you make a matching sound?' Groups are challenged to plan an imaginative holiday idea, and then perform it with accompanying sound.

b practise, improve and refine performance. The last lesson of the year gives greater freedom to the pupils in the decision-making and organisation of their practising. It is hoped that the created actions and sounds will be surprising, humorous and varied, a tribute to their enthusiasm, energy and 'togetherness' as a class, and an enjoyable climax to the year's programme.

c make simple judgements about others' performances to improve the accuracy, quality and variety of the performance. From Year 3 onwards, observers should have been trained to value demonstrations; be appreciative and sensitive observers; express pleasure and encouragement when evaluating achievements; and make helpful comments regarding areas that might be improved.

Warm-up Activities

1–2 The teacher decides and leads the class in the few, varied actions to be done by everyone. The class, copying the actions, then add in the vocal sounds that fit these actions.

Movement Skills Training

1 One partner is asked to start making small, smooth, continuous movements on the spot. The other partner, standing a metre away, is asked to accompany the small actions with vocal sounds that are equally smooth and continuous, and at the right rhythm as an accompaniment.

2 The mover changes to less predictable, bigger, more angular and even robotic actions, still on the spot. A bigger, jerkier, louder vocal-sound accompaniment is required.

3 The inclusion of speed and body height changes by the mover is a final challenge for the sound person, who has to change the speeds and intensity of the rising and falling sounds.

4–5 Partners change places and the new movement-making partner performs on the move, travelling slowly and predictably; then more unpredictably and robotically; then with more variety of speed and level, accompanied by the travelling, sound-making partner.

6 The half-watching-half demonstrations focus on both the impressive range of actions and the quality and variety of the sound making.

Voice Sounds Dance

1–7 A holidays 'Voice Sounds' dance focuses on actions, places and food associated with being on holiday. The class practise examples of holiday actions, place names and foods, saying and elongating and shortening the descriptive words, and accompanying them with body movements whose speeds change with the speed of the spoken words. Travelling is the easiest ongoing accompaniment to parts of spoken words. A sudden jump and landing can speed up a part of a word. Turning, rising and falling are also good ways to slowly elongate parts of a name, sport or a food. A quick gesture of arms, shoulders or head can be surprising. Good teams of five will include all of these plus a still team ending.

Games

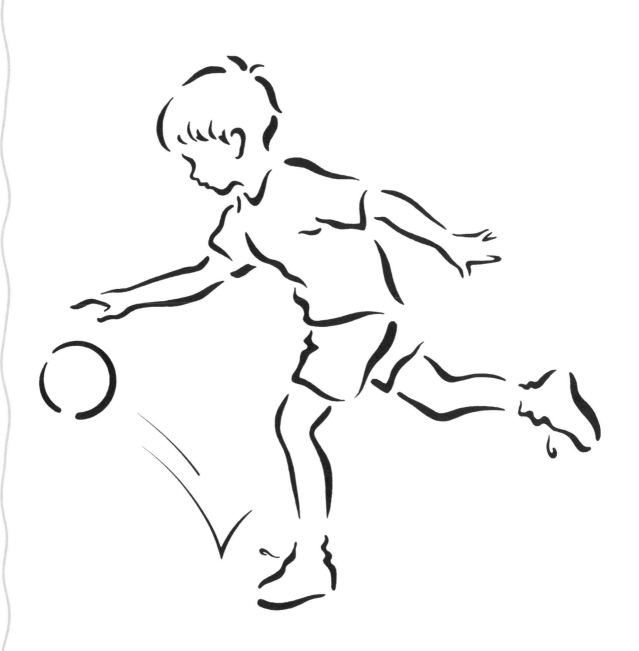

Introduction To Games

Individual and team games are part of our national heritage and an essential part of the physical education programme. Skills learned during games lend themselves to being practised away from school, alone or with friends or parents, and are the skills most likely to be used in participating in worthwhile physical and social activities long after leaving school – an important, long-term aim of physical education.

Vigorous, whole body activity in the fresh air promotes normal, healthy growth and physical development, stimulating the heart, lungs and big muscle groups, particularly the legs. Games lessons come nearest of all physical education activities to demonstrating what we understand by the expression 'children at play'. Pupils are involved in play-like, exciting, adventurous chasing and dodging as they try to outwit opponents in games and competitive activities. Such close, friendly 'combat' with others can help to compensate for the increasingly isolated, over-protected, self-absorbed nature of much of today's childhood.

All the lessons in this book are planned for the playground where most primary school games teaching now takes place. Precious time spent travelling to a field; the high cost of coach travel; a wet, muddy surface for much of the year; the need for expensive footwear; and a playing surface on which it is difficult to practise the variety of activities and small-sided games we need to offer, have all combined to make the school's own playground the preferred setting for the games programme.

Each rectangular third of the netball court is clearly marked with painted lines that should last for several years. These thirds are an ideal size for the three different games that are the climax of each lesson. It is recommended that schools have a line painted from end line to end line, in a different colour to ensure that the netball court is not affected. The extra line means that each rectangle is sub-divided into two halves. The line can be the centre for games across each third and a useful, definite marking for those games, where, for example, you may want to limit defenders or attackers to their own halves. The line can also be a 'net' for summer term games of short-tennis, quoits or volleyball.

The playground 'classroom' rectangle is essential because it contains the whole class in a limited space within which the teacher can see, and be easily seen and heard by, the whole class, and it prevents accidents by keeping the class well away from potential hazards such as concrete seats, hutted classrooms, fences or walls, all of which should be several metres outside the games rectangle.

Games will appeal to, and be very popular with the majority if: the pupils are always moving; the games are exciting; nobody is left doing nothing; they are fun to play; there is plenty of action; and if rules prevent quarrels, let the game run smoothly, let everyone have a turn, and prevent foul play.

The following monthly lesson plans and accompanying explanatory notes are designed to help teachers and schools with ideas for lessons that progress from month to month, and from year to year. Each lesson is repeated three or four times to allow plenty of time for planning, practising, repeating and improving. The plans also aim to provide a focus for staffroom togetherness and unity of purpose regarding the programme's aims, content, teaching methods, standards, and expectations of levels of achievement.

The Games Lesson Plan for Juniors – 30–45 minutes

All of the lessons that follow are designed for the school playground where most primary school games teaching takes place. Each rectangular third of the netball court is an ideal size for the three different, small-sided games or group practices which are the climax of each lesson.

Warm-up and Footwork Practices (4–6 minutes) start the lesson and aim to get the class quickly into action, and stimulate vigorous leg muscle activity which, in turn, stimulates the heart and lungs. Pupils enjoy practising running, jumping, chasing, dodging, marking, changing speed and direction, side-stepping, swerving and accelerating. Older juniors learn correct stopping and starting so that footwork rules in netball and basketball are understood. 'Faking' by moving head, shoulder or foot to one side, then suddenly moving the opposite way; sprint and change of direction dodges; and offensive and defensive footwork, used in 'one against one' dodges, are all practised.

Skills Practices (8–12 minutes) form the middle part of the lesson with the whole class using the same implement and practising the same skills so that the teaching and coaching applies to everyone. With younger, less experienced pupils, the practices include individual then partner practices of skills they might have performed before. They progress on to co-operative and competitive, partner and small group practices of skills already experienced to make practising more like the games situation.

Invent a Game or Skill Practice (3–5 minutes) provides pupils with the opportunity to plan a practice that further develops the skills featured in the middle part of the lesson, or to invent their own game complete with agreed rules and scoring systems.

Group Practices and Small-sided Games (15–22 minutes) can provide one of the most eagerly anticipated parts of all junior school physical education. They are the climax of the lesson and must be started promptly to allow their full time allocation. One of the three games or activities always includes use of the implement and skills practised in the middle part of the lesson. The three games or group practices take part in the thirds of the netball court. If a second court is available, it can be used for any activity that benefits from a bigger playing pitch. The three sets of implements to be used will have been placed adjacent to, but outside, the enclosed rectangles where they will be used.

The main organisational challenge is explaining and starting this final part of the lesson on the first day of a new series of lessons. At the start of the year, the six mixed teams or groups will have been chosen and given 'Your starting place for games and group activities.' If the teacher explains only one game at a time to the ten about to play it, the remaining twenty will be standing, losing heat and patience, and often becoming noisy and inattentive.

The answer is to have all three groups playing the same game or practice, one of the three to be introduced. Instructions about scoring, the main rules and method of re-starting after a score, will apply to all. The signal 'Start!' applies to everyone. When all three games are being played and are obviously understood, the teacher moves to and teaches one group its planned game or activity. When this group is going well, the teacher moves on to and teaches a second group its planned activity. The teacher then says 'Stop, everyone, and look at each of the two games or activities some of you have not seen yet.' Each new game or activity is demonstrated with an accompanying commentary from the teacher. The three groups then rotate on to their second activity, and finally to their third and last activity.

A Pattern for Teaching a Games Skill or Practice

Excellent lesson 'pace' is expressed in almost non-stop activity with no bad behaviour stoppages and no 'dead spots' caused by queues, over-long explanations or too many time-consuming demonstrations. The teaching of each of the skills combining to make a games lesson determines the quality of the lesson's pace – a main feature of an excellent physical education lesson.

A typical games lesson with its warm-up and footwork practices, skills practices, and small-sided group practices and games, will have about a dozen skills. Whatever the skill, there is a pattern for teaching it.

1   **Quickly into action**. In a few words, explain the task, and challenge the class to start. 'Can you stand, two big steps apart, and throw and catch the small ball to your partner for a two-handed catch?' If a short demonstration is needed, the teacher can work with a pupil who has been alerted. Class practice should start quickly after the five seconds it took the teacher to make the challenge.

2   **Emphasise the main teaching points, one at a time, while the class is working**. z A well-behaved class does not need to be stopped to listen to the next point. 'Hold both hands forward to show your partner where to aim.' 'Watch the ball into your cupped hands.'

3   **Identify and praise good work, while the class is working**. Comments are heard by all; remind the class of key points; and inspire the praised to even greater effort. 'Well done, Sarah and Daniel. You are throwing and catching at the right height and speed, and watching the ball into your hands.'

4   **Teach for individual improvement while class are working**. 'Liam, hold both hands forward to give Lucy a still target to aim at.' 'Chloe and Ben, stand closer. You are too far apart.'

5   **A demonstration can be used**, briefly, to show good quality or an example of what is required. 'Stop everyone, please, and watch how Ravinder and Michael let their hands "give" as they receive the ball, to stop it bouncing out again.' Less than twelve seconds later, all resume practising, understanding what 'giving hands' means.

6   **Very occasionally, to avoid taking too much activity time, a short demonstration can be followed by comments**. 'Stop and watch Leroy and Emily. Tell me what makes their throwing and catching so smooth and accurate.' The class watch about six throws and three or four comments are invited. For example, 'They are nicely balanced with one foot forward.' 'Their hands are well forward, to take the ball early, then give, smoothly and gently.'

7   **Thanks are given to performers and those making helpful comments**. Further practice takes place with reminders of the good things seen and commented on.

Progressing a Games Lesson over 4 or 5 Lessons

Gymnastic activities and dance lessons can begin at a simple level of performing the actions neatly, because they are natural and easy. The challenge for the teacher and class is then to plan and develop movement sequences that link these natural actions together, and refine them by adding 'movement elements' such as changes of speed, direction, shape and tension.

Developing a games lesson is different from the above because the eventual target is the mastery of the specific games skills included in the lesson. Such skills include:

❍ good footwork used in stopping, starting, changing direction, chasing after and dodging away from other players

❍ sending, receiving and travelling with a ball in invasion, striking/fielding and net games, and controlling other games implements such as skipping ropes, quoits, rackets, hoops and bean bags

❍ inventing games with agreed rules in co-operation with a partner or small group. Fairness, safety, lots of action and an understanding of the need for rules are the intended outcomes

❍ playing competitive games as individuals, with partners, and in small-sided games

❍ understanding the skills and particular roles of players as they attack and defend in the three types of games.

Often the starting point, practising the new skill, is a problem, because controlling the implement is difficult. Balls, bats, hoops, skipping ropes, rackets, quoits and bean bags behave unpredictably and the teacher has to simplify the planned skills to enable pupils to succeed and progress in subsequent lessons. Reception class pupils, for example, might have to walk beside a partner, handing the bean bag to each other, before progressing to throwing and catching. In a Junior school, 2 versus 1 throwing and catching practice, the teacher can ask the defending pupil in the middle to be passive, with arms down at sides, not aiming to 'steal' the ball that is being passed, and only keeping between the two passing players to make them move sideways and forwards, into a good space to receive the ball.

The varied skills headings listed, fit neatly into both infant and junior games lessons, with their:

❍ footwork practices

❍ skills practices, which can include 'invent a game'

❍ group practices and small-sided games, which can include 'invent a game' and challenges to suggest ways to improve a game with a new rule, other ways to score, or limits on player movement.

Step by step, revising the previous lesson's work, and introducing only one teaching point at a time, the teacher progresses one of the skills of the lesson, for example:

1   Try the slow overhead pull of the rope as it slides along the ground towards you.

2   Can you travel, running over the sliding rope, one foot after the other? Which is your leading leg?

3   On the spot, try a jump and bounce for each turn of the rope. (Slow '1 and, 2 and' skipping action.)

4   Try slow running over the rope. Use a small, turning wrist action with hands out wide at waist height.

5   Skip from space to space. Then show me skipping in each space.

6   On the spot, try the slow double beat and the quicker single beat. Then show me neat, non-stop skipping.

7   Pretend your group is on a stage, all doing your best skipping.

Invasion Games for Juniors – the Excitement of Competition

Outwitting one or more opponents – stages in progressing the level of competition

Stage 1 Offensive footwork practices without a ball – starting, stopping, changing direction, accelerating, sprinting, dodging, pivoting, feinting with head, foot or shoulder.

1 Jog, looking for spaces, when near others. Sprint suddenly when you have lots of room.

2 Run freely and change direction on 'Change!'

3 Practise side steps on to new line, still facing the same way.

Stage 2 Co-operative practices with a partner – dodges, direction changes, side steps, body fakes, changes of speed, and helpful comments from following, encouraging partner.

1 Follow your leader who will try dodges to lose you. Follower comments on the dodging.

2 Follow the leader who suddenly sprints to lose you, by speed and direction changes. Follower comments on which was the more successful – speed or direction changes.

3 Jog, side by side, at same speed. Leader does a sudden sprint to be free for a moment.

4 Partners face each other, one metre apart. Attacking partner progresses forward with small, rapid steps to try to make defender lose the 'in line' position between attacker and target line.

Stage 3 Competitive practices with a partner – gives 'attacking' player practice in checking the success of his or her repertoire of offensive dodges.

1 'Tag' where dodger tries to avoid being touched by chaser, who then becomes the dodger.

2 Dodge and Mark. Marker tries to stay within touching distance of dodger on teacher's 'Stop!'

3 One against one, across court, using body feints, plus direction and speed changes.

Stage 4 Offensive footwork practices with a partner, using a ball – trying to reach goal line with ball still in possession in dribbling games such as hockey, football or basketball. These little games need only a short stretch of line as a 'goal' with a 5 metre approach to this line.

1 Teacher allocates a number of minutes for each to attack from a start position 5 metres back. An attack ends when goal is scored, defender takes possession, or ball goes out of area.

2 In '3 lives' games, the same attacker starts three times, then changes roles.

Stage 5 Two against two practices with a ball – two kinds.
1 '3 lives', with same pair attacking three times from a 5 metre approach. After the three turns as attackers are used up, attackers become defenders.

2 End-to-end games across a third of the court with both teams trying to score. Passive defending, with the defending pair marking and keeping 'in line', but not tackling, encourages a flowing, enjoyable game for the less experienced.

Stage 6 Playing 3-, 4- or 5-a-side games – including scaled-down netball, hockey, basketball, football, handball, rugby touch, and created games such as heading ball, skittleball and hoop ball.

1 Attackers ideally understand – 'Pass and move!' 'Give and go to be available!'

2 A named team-mate moves to opponents' line as 'target player' to receive or give passes.

3 'Fast break' every time your team steals possession when none of your team is marked.

National Curriculum Requirements for Games – Key Stage 2: the Main Features

'The government believes that two hours of physical activity a week, including the National Curriculum for Physical Education and extra-curricular activities, should be an aspiration for all schools. This applies to all key stages.'

Programme of study   Pupils should be taught to:

a   play and make up small-sided and modified competitive net, striking/fielding and invasion games
b   use skills and tactics and apply basic principles suitable for attacking and defending
c   work with others to organise and keep the games going.

Attainment target   Pupils should be able to demonstrate that they can:

a   select and use skills, actions and ideas appropriately, applying them with co-ordination and control
b   when performing, draw on what they know about tactics and strategy
c   compare and comment on skills and ideas used in own work by modifying and refining skills and techniques.

Main NC headings when considering assessment, progression and expectation

○   **Planning**, with pupils being challenged to think ahead carefully about their intended responses;

○   **Performing and improving performance** expressed in safe, focused, hard work by attentive pupils who continually aim for a more skilful and confident performance;

○   **Linking actions** smoothly and safely, using space sensibly, and able to remember and repeat the whole sequence successfully from its start right through to its controlled finish;

○   **Reflecting and making judgements** to help pupils progress and improve, as they plan again, adapting and altering as required, guided by their own and others' comments and judgements.

Achievement and progression

One way of assessing how pupils are progressing is by referring to the main requirements within the NC, under the following three headings:

Planning – Performing and participating in a thoughtful, well-organised way is the result of good planning, which takes place before and during performance. Subsequent performances will be influenced by the planning that also takes place after reflecting on the success or otherwise of the activity. Where planning standards are considered to be satisfactory, there is evidence of: (a) thinking ahead to visualise the finished action; (b) good judgements and decisions being made; (c) good understanding of what is required; (d) originality and variety through trying own ideas; (e) consideration for others, sharing space and equipment well; (f) positive qualities such as enthusiasm, wholeheartedness and the capacity for working and practising hard to achieve.

Performing and improving performance – We are fortunate in Physical Education because of the visual nature of the activities. It is easy to see, note and remember how pupils perform, demonstrating skill and versatility. Where standards of performing are satisfactory there is evidence of: (a) neatness, accuracy and 'correctness'; (b) skilfulness and versatility; (c) consistency and the ability to remember and repeat; (d) appropriateness of responses and safe, successful outcomes; (e) originality of solutions; (f) ability to do more than one thing at a time, linking a series of actions with increasing fluency, accuracy, control and skill; (g) adaptability and ability to make sudden adjustments as needed; (h) pleasure from participation; (i) a clear understanding of what was required.

Evaluating/reflecting – Evaluation is intended to inform further planning and preparation by helping both performers and spectators with guidance and ideas for altering, adapting, extending and improving performances. Where standards in evaluating are satisfactory, pupils are able to: (a) observe accurately; (b) identify the parts of a performance that they liked; (c) pick out the main features being demonstrated; (d) make comparisons between two performances; (e) reflect on the accuracy of the work; (f) comment on the quality of the movement, using simple terms; (g) suggest ways in which the work might be improved; (h) express pleasure in a performance.

Year 5 Games Programme

Pupils should be able to:

Autumn	Spring	Summer
1 Respond quickly; accept rules; wear sensible clothing.	1 Encourage good sporting behaviour when playing, refining own games, considering rules, scoring, tactics.	1 Practise to improve skills of net and striking/fielding games with a partner or small group in a games situation.
2 Send, receive and travel with a ball with increasing control and accuracy.	2 Send, receive and travel with a ball with greater confidence and control.	2 Demonstrate overarm bowling action from standing and after a run up.
3 Refine and apply dodging and marking techniques in games.	3 Show adaptability, using one- and two-handed, varied passes.	3 Field ball with confidence from varied speeds, heights, lengths, and throw in at speed.
4 Mark player with and without the ball, denying space.	4 Value good footwork in offence (side-steps, quick stops, direction and speed changes) and defence (marking 'in line').	4 Demonstrate forehand and backhand volleys with confidence.
5 Develop habitual use of 'Pass and follow'; 'Give and go'; and 'Move to receive a pass.'	5 Mark an opponent, with and without the ball, frustrating his or her movement.	5 Co-operate to make long rallies with a partner.
6 Plan ways to keep small-sided games moving and involving everyone.	6 Learn to 'screen' a ball fairly from a chasing opponent.	6 Show ability to draw partner into net by varying length of strike.
7 Collect a ball on the run with confidence and control with hands, feet or stick.	7 Experience many small-sided versions of recognised games – football, hockey, rugby, netball, basketball, as well as benchball, headingball and team passing.	7 Decide on rules, scoring, player limits to keep games flowing and involve everyone fairly.
8 Work co-operatively with team-mates to work ball from end to end.	8 Apply basic principles of attack – keep possession, support ball carrier, create space, often by keeping out of the way.	8 Condemn anti-social behaviour, including unfair play.
9 In small-sided versions of recognised games, revise common skills and principles of attack and defence, e.g. quick passing 'fast break' if possible; mark 'in line' in 'one-on-one' defending.	9 Apply basic principles of defence – mark opponent, try interceptions, deny space.	9 Observe partner's volleying and suggest how to improve.
10 Be able to watch a team's defence or attack and comment on its effectiveness.	10 Use simple tactics like shaping a team attack to make space.	10 Experience small-sided versions of cricket, tennis, volleyball, rounders, adapting them to include everyone.
	11 Be able to explain a successful team or group demonstration.	11 Compare two performances and point out differences in content and effectiveness.
		12 Reflect on the physical and social benefits of a good Games programme and whole-hearted participation.

Lesson Plan 1 • 30-45 minutes
September

Warm-up and Footwork Practices
4–6 minutes

1 Show me your best running, quiet and not following anyone. Can you visit all parts of our playground 'classroom' – sides, ends, middle and corners?

2 Keep running, and when I call 'Stop!' let me see who is first and last, standing perfectly still and balanced on tiptoes on a line. Stop! Repeat.

Skills Practices: with small balls
8–12 minutes

Individual practices

1 Walk or jog, throwing ball from one hand to the other.

2 Walk, throwing ball up, clap hands, catch with both hands.

3 Juggle ball to keep it bouncing up and down, using hands, feet, thighs, head, etc. Keep your best score.

Partner practices

1 Stand close, about 2 metres apart, and throw to each other. Each move back 1 large step and repeat. Move back, repeat. After 4 or 5 moves, start coming in again.

2 Stand 3–4 metres apart. One throws straight to partner, who returns it with bounce half way. Change over after 6.

Invent a Game or Practice in 2s
3–5 minutes

Can you and your partner invent a game or practice with 1 small ball, throwing, catching or aiming? You can use part of a line if you wish, and no more than 1 third of the netball court. (For example, aiming practice at a line between you, starting 1 metre back from the line. Move back 1 step each time to see what is the limit of your accurate aiming.)

Group Practices and Small-sided Games
15–22 minutes

Small ball between 2

Dribbling ball by hand or foot, screening ball from pursuing partner (illustrated). Decide on 1 rule to give pursuer a fair chance.

Hand-tennis

2 with 2, rope 'net' tied between netball posts. See how long you can keep rally going over rope 'net'.

Competition in pairs

Rotate clockwise, 3 shots each. Netball, hockey, football and basketball shooting.

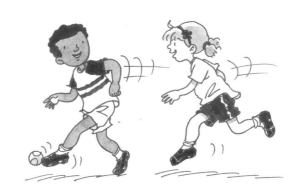

Games

Teaching notes and NC guidance
Development over 4–5 lessons

Lesson's main emphases:

a the NC general requirement to respond readily to instructions, and to be physically active;

b re-establishing the good habits and traditions of: good, safe and unselfish spacing with no uncalled-for talking; whole-hearted participation with all contributing to the 'scene of busy activity', essential and obvious in all good lessons.

Equipment: 30 small balls; long rope 'net' tied between 2 netball posts; 4 cones for goals; 2 hockey sticks; 2 large balls for football and basketball shooting.

Warm-up and Footwork Practices

1 Pursue the elusive 'correct', quiet, easy running style with its lifting of heels, knees, arms, shoulders and head. Encourage running along straight lines, not the whole class following each other anti-clockwise as is common in primary schools.

2 The first-to-stop-on-a-line game is a way of training the class to be listening while working, as well as providing for the 'quick decision-making' needs within the NC.

Skills Practices: with small balls

Individual practices

1 In controlling the small ball, throwing and catching, the main point is to watch the ball closely all the time, catch it in a sensible position near eye level, and let the body parts concerned 'feel' how much effort is needed. Too much force in throwing, batting and kicking is a common fault.

2 The hand-clap places both hands in a good place and shape for a catch, near eye level where you can see ball well.

3 Allow 1 bounce between hits with the varied body parts. You need to 'keep on your toes' to move quickly to the next bouncing place, to be balanced, ready.

Partner practices

1 2–5 metres apart, partners should be throwing underarm, aiming at each other's hands reaching out to where they want the throw to go. Thrower follows through after sending the ball. Catcher lets hands 'give' after the catch.

2 The throw to bounce ball about 1 metre in front of partner starts from above shoulder.

Invent a Game or Practice in 2s

The example suggested can be co-operative, with pair keeping best score of consecutive hits, or competitive, trying to beat partner's number of hits.

Group Practices and small-sided Games

Small ball between 2

The 1 versus 1 dribbling to screen the ball is competitive. Come to an agreement on the size of the 'pitch' to give chaser a chance, and 1 main rule for fairness.

Hand-tennis

In hand-tennis, emphasise 'side on to your partner' when you hit the ball at ideally just below shoulder height.

Competition in pairs

Careful, well-placed shots in hockey and football, rather than over-hard shots that send the ball out of court and play.

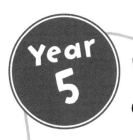

Year 5

Lesson Plan 2 • 30-45 minutes
October

Warm-up and Footwork Practices
4—6 minutes

1   Follow your leader, who will show you a sequence of 2 or 3 lively leg actions. Can you work together to repeat the actions in unison?

2   Half of the class with coloured bands tucked into back of shorts. All chase to collect and retain as many bands as possible.

Skills Practices: with large balls
8—12 minutes

1   About 3 metres apart, practise passing to your partner's chest and then running into a new space to receive the return pass. Use 2-handed, chest, bounce and overhead passes.

2   Run side by side, interpass rugby fashion.

3   Shadow dribbling with foot. Change after 6 touches. Following partner notes the actions being shown and changes places with leader to try to repeat the sequence.

Invent a Game or Practice
3—5 minutes

Can you invent a game for 4 players and 1 ball, using 1 or more of the 3 ball skills above? (For example, 3 versus 1, where the '3' may keep the ball by using chest passes when a partner is available, or football dribbling when no partner is available.)

Group Practices and Small-sided Games
15—22 minutes

2 v 2 passing large ball

3 passes = 1 goal. Encourage short passes to partner, who should have moved into a space (illustrated).

Floor-football

4 or 5 a side. To score, arrive on opponents' goal line, ball under foot. Keep ball below knee height. Receive, look for team-mate, pass, move to new space to help. Decide ways to make game more 'open', for example 2 players in front half, 2 in rear.

Free-netball

No positions or limits on who may shoot. Passing to a partner who has moved, unmarked, into new space. 'Pass and follow your pass. Stop shouting for a pass. Move to a good space to be ready to receive a pass.'

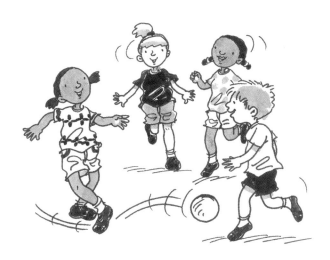

Games

Teaching notes and NC guidance
Development over 4–5 lessons

Lesson's main emphases:

a the NC requirements to improve the skills of sending, receiving and travelling with a ball, and to make appropriate decisions quickly and plan their responses;

b remembering that with the approach of colder weather, the habit of quiet work, immediate responses and near non-stop activity must be insisted upon so that all keep warm, and all parts of an enjoyable and varied lesson can be covered.

Equipment: 15 large balls; 15 coloured bands; 1 flattish large ball for the floor-football; 1 set netball apparatus.

Warm-up and Footwork Practices

1 In follow-the-leader, emphasise that leader must lead partner into good spaces, visiting all parts of the playground, preferably travelling along straight lines. 3 actions would be a challenging sequence to observe and copy.

2 In coloured-band-chase, let us be adventurous and do more chasing after others' bands than hiding to retain own band.

Skills Practices: with large balls

1 3 metres apart, 'Pass and move sideways into a space. Give ball and go. Pass, move, signalling with leading hand, receive' until these become habitual actions over a short distance.

2 Only 1–2 metres apart in side-by-side rugby-style passing and catching. Turn the upper body and pass ball with both hands just ahead of partner for him to run on to.

3 Shadow dribbling, follow leader who peels off to end of line after a short sequence, using changes of feet or direction.

Invent a Game or Practice

1 ball among 4 to create an activity, competitive or co-operative, to develop and improve any of the 3 skills already practised. If a group has no idea, suggest the 3 versus 1 sample practice.

Group Practices and Small-sided Games

2 v 2 passing large ball

In 2-versus-2 team passing, defending pair can be passive (not trying to grab ball) if passers are being unsuccessful. Whether passive or highly active, 1 defender must confront the ball-carrier, keeping between him and the intended receiver. This forces the receiver to move quickly to find a space not blocked by the ball-handler's defender.

Floor-football

Softish football stays in playing area better than a hard bouncer, giving more action and less waiting about. Scoring is difficult and the defending team has a big advantage. Limits may need to be put on the defenders (no tackling in opponents' half, for example).

Free-netball

In netball, encourage shooting with a point for a near miss, hitting ring, and 2 points for a correct score. Emphasise that the passer is expected to move 2–3 metres into a space, to be available to receive the next pass.

Lesson Plan 3 • 30-45 minutes
November

Warm-up and Footwork Practices
4–6 minutes

1   Run, changing direction often. Pushing hard with 1 foot to go other way.

2   Teacher's-space tag. Try to cross middle third of netball court, guarded by teacher and 4 helpers in coloured bands, without being caught. Crossing untouched earns you 1 point. (Teacher checks best score and changes helpers frequently.)

Skills Practices: with hockey sticks and balls
8–12 minutes

Individual practices

1   Revise running with stick in right hand 'carry' position. On 'Change!' bring left hand to top of stick, stick down to just above ground. On next 'Change!' return stick to 1 hand in suitcase position at right side.

2   Indian dribble side to side, along a line, around chalk marks, or around cones or quoits. Hold flat side of stick against right side of ball, stick head pointing up. Now point head down and transfer to other, left hand side of ball. Move ball left and right with stick head pointing up and down.

Partner practice

Dribble about 4 metres to line between you. Push to partner who receives and repeats. Run back to own line after passing.

Invent a Game or Skills Practice
3–5 minutes

Invent a game in 2s with 1 ball and part of line, using dribble and/or gentle push pass. (For example, stationary partner passes ball to running partner, who moves to left and right to receive and return. Aim at space into which running partner is moving.)

Group Practices and Small-sided Games
15–22 minutes

2 v 2 hockey across half of area

Attacking pair interpass to place ball on opponents' line. Opponents may only intercept a pass. Push-pass gently. No tackling. When opponent confronts you, you must pass to partner.

Bench-ball

4 or 5 a side. Goal scored when catcher on chalk 'bench' receives good throw. Change catcher often, particularly in cold weather. Encourage 'pass and move to receive a pass'.

Heading-ball

Large foam ball, 4 or 5 a side. Goal scored when attacker heads ball over opponents' line. No running with ball. Pass and run forwards. When near line expect pass to forehead for shot at goal. After a goal, ball thrown in from end line by team scored against.

Games

Teaching notes and NC guidance
Development over 4–5 lessons

Lesson's main emphases:

a   the NC requirements to explore and understand the common skills and principles, including attack and defence, of invasion games, to sustain energetic activity and show understanding of what is happening to their bodies when they are exercising.

b   in really cold weather keep the discussion, which ideally follows every demonstration, until back in the classroom. A class trained to expect questions in the warm after being outside will watch more intently, remember and, of course, learn, which is the whole point.

Equipment: 30 hockey sticks and small balls; 1 large ball and 1 large foam ball; playground chalk for marking the 'bench'.

Warm-up and Footwork Practices

1   Practise direction changes at lines, with right foot, for example, stopping you then pushing off to the left.

2   In teacher's-space tag, emphasise careful running and dodging, looking out for others. Use good dodges, not dangerous fast sprints, to avoid being caught. Stop the game every 12 seconds to keep careful control, calm them all down, and bring in new chasers.

Skills Practices: with hockey sticks and balls

Individual practices

1   Running, carrying stick at right side, is a good exercise in 'sustaining energetic activity' as well as a good teaching point, practising the efficient, safe way to run with the stick when not playing the ball.

2   In side-to-side dribbling, strong left-hand grip turns the stick, which rotates inside the sleeve of the more loosely held right hand. 'Point of stick up, point of stick down. To left, to right.'

Partner practice

In the push, emphasise that the stick is placed behind the ball then pushed, with no sound of stick on ball, not hit with a big, dangerous, preliminary backswing.

Invent a Game or Skills Practice

If the less creative are having difficulty in devising and agreeing a practice, and are standing, becoming cold, they should have the example activity given to them to do.

Group Practices and Small-sided Games

2 v 2 hockey across half of area

In hockey, dribble to advance the ball until confronted by an opponent when you must pass the ball, ideally into a space for partner to run in to. Players may attack side by side or one ahead of the other.

Bench-ball

In bench-ball, only the catcher may stand on the 'bench'. After a goal, the team scored against throw in from the end line. Bench-catcher is encouraged to move from side to side along the bench to assist throwers in finding him, unmarked, still on the bench.

Heading-ball

In heading-ball, 2 players are needed to make a goal. You may not throw the ball up and head it yourself.

Lesson Plan 4 • 30-45 minutes
December

Warm-up and Footwork Practices
4—6 minutes

1   Run around the whole netball court once, then run a third, hop a third, and leap a third to one end. Repeat.

2   Dodge and mark in 2s. Marker shadows dodger. On 'Stop!' both must stop immediately to see who is the winner – dodger clear or marker still within touching distance. Change duties.

Skills Practices: with rugby balls or large balls
8—12 minutes

Group practices in 3s with 1 ball

1   Passing weave. A passes to B and goes to B's position. B runs to centre with ball, passes to C, then goes to C's position as C runs into centre to pass to A. Receive; run in and pass to opposite side; run to outside.

2   2 v 1 team passing. 2 passers try to make groups of 4 passes, which equal a goal. '2s' keep about 3 metres apart only to give '1' a chance.

Invent a Game or Skills Practice
3—5 minutes

Invent a game in 3s with 1 ball and part of line in small area of playground. Use dodging and passing. (For example, passing pair try to touch third person with ball. When touched, you become one of chasing pair who must pass and not run with ball.)

Group Practices and Small-sided Games
15—22 minutes

Rugby-touch

4 or 5 a side. Place ball on opponents' line to score. After score, opponents throw in ball from behind their line. With ball, run forwards and straight. Pass if touched. Increase scoring chances with target player on line for passes.

Mini-basketball

4 or 5 a side, netball apparatus. Left and right side forwards and defenders keep to own sides of court for more open game. You may dribble, but passing is quicker. In attack, a diamond shape with target player near opponents' goal is a useful tactic.

Playground-hockey

4 or 5 a side. Score by placing ball on opponents' goal line (illustrated). Left and right side attackers anddefenders keep to own side of court so more room to move and pass. Push-pass only. No hitting or swinging stick behind or in front.

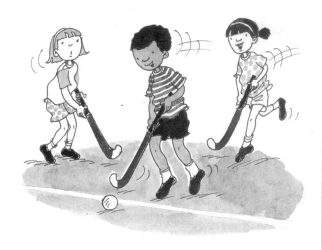

Teaching notes and NC guidance
Development over 4–5 lessons

Lesson's main emphases:

a   the NC requirement to play small-sided and simplified versions of recognised games.

b   taking a reasonable level of individual and partner skill for granted now that we are half way through Year 5 of the NC, and moving on to a higher level of team thinking and performing. 'Watch this team' or 'Watch this group' should now be heard as often as 'Watch this individual' or 'Watch this pair'. The team, the game, the offence, the defence, the tactics, the rules and the scoring systems are all now to be emphasised more as we set and demand higher standards and levels of expectation during these primary school years of enthusiastic pursuit of skilfulness and achievement.

Equipment: 10 large or rugby balls; netball apparatus and 1 large ball; 10 hockey sticks and a playground-hockey ball.

Warm-up and Footwork Practices

1   Whole class start behind an end line. All run around the outside of the court and back to starting line, from which they then progress down court with running, then hopping, then long stride leaping. Repeat, starting from opposite end line.

2   In dodge-and-mark, emphasise 'Use good dodges, direction and speed changes, and fakes with head, foot or shoulder to dodge away, not high-speed sprinting which can cause bumps and accidents and gives no practice in either dodging or marking.'

Skills Practices: with rugby balls or large balls

Group practices in 3s with 1 ball

1   In 3-player passing-weave, ball starts at centre, from where it is thrown to an outside person who runs, carrying ball in to centre, for next pass out to opposite side. After each pass you follow to the place where you passed and all 3 players will be moving, almost non-stop, as they weave around the figure 8.

2   2 versus 1, where '2s' may not run with ball, and work hard to move into spaces to which passes can be made. Pass across 2–3 metres only, since long throws mean the '1' in the middle has no chance to make an interception.

Invent a Game or Skills Practice

Another example might be for the '1' in a 2 versus 1 game to try to touch the ball, then change places with the one who had the ball, becoming one of the ball-passing players.

Group Practices and Small-sided Games

Rugby-touch

In rugby-touch, the 'tackle' has to be made by both hands of tackler touching the runner's hips. This is harder to achieve than the previous touch of hand on person, helps the attacking team and leads to more scoring if runners will keep on running.

Mini-basketball

In mini-basketball, aim for a '1 on 1' marking situation, where each knows his opponent to mark or dodge away from.

Playground-hockey

In playground-hockey, restrict player movement in an agreed way to allow more open play. Outlaw and make big fuss against hitting.

Lesson Plan 5 • 30–45 minutes
January

Warm-up and Footwork Practices
4–6 minutes

1   In your running, practise side-steps and direction changes to avoid others coming towards you.

2   1-versus-1, across-court, line-to-line dodging and marking, with dodger using good footwork and fakes. Change duties.

Skills Practices: with large balls
8–12 minutes

Partner practices

1   2-hand pass from shoulder over running partner's head for a jump and catch, about 3 metres away. Run to space to jump to catch.

2   Juggle ball with foot, thigh or head. Single, controlled bouncing between you both.

3   1 versus 1, dribbling with foot to screen ball from pursuing partner.

Invent a Game
3–5 minutes

Can you invent a 1-versus-1 game, using the throwing, juggling or screening practised above? (For example, football-tennis over a line 'net'.)

Group Practices and Small-sided Games
15–22 minutes

Team passing

4 or 5 a side, 1 large ball. Pass to team-mate in a space and not too far from you, ideally about 3 metres. Grab ball into stomach on receipt. 4 good passes = 1 goal. Vary passes to include chest, bounce and overhead passes.

Free-netball

4 or 5 a side (illustrated). No limits to area or who may shoot. No dribbling. Pass and move forwards for return pass. 1 point for near miss, hitting hoop. 2 points for goal, through hoop. If overcrowding around ball, discuss solutions (for example, at least 1 to stay in own half).

Floor-football

4 or 5 a side, slightly flat ball. Score by arriving on opponents' goal line, ball under foot. Keep ball below knee height. Defenders stay in own half, attackers in opponents' half, so less overcrowding. To encourage passing, 2 passes may be made before opponents can tackle.

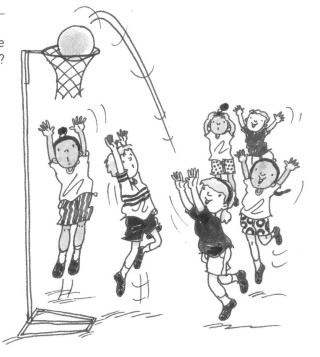

Games

Teaching notes and NC guidance
Development over 4–5 lessons

Lesson's main emphases:

a the NC requirements to plan, practise, improve and refine performance, including within their own created games with their rules and scoring systems.

b remembering that mid-winter and dark evenings probably mean that the lifestyle of the majority of our girls and boys is now at its least physical, most inactive and sedentary, and mostly indoors. This lively lesson, out in the fresh air, with its chasing-game warm-up, varied co-operative and competitive skills practices, 'invent a game' and varied small-sided team games, aims to inspire the action, play, fun and friendly competition that is particularly lacking in January.

Equipment: 15 large balls; netball apparatus; 1 flattish big or medium sized ball for football.

Warm-up and Footwork Practices

1 The side-steps and direction change practices could be done in two-thirds or one-third of the netball court so that you would continually be dodging others coming towards you.

2 In 1-versus-1, across-court, line-to-line dodge-and-mark, ask the dodgers to move fairly slowly and try to beat the defender with a sudden clever dodge or direction change, never a sprint past them.

Skills Practices: with large balls

Partner practices

1 Runner moves when thrower signals readiness by bringing ball up to throwing position. Runner can also signal by pointing 1 arm to side chosen.

2 You can juggle to a pattern. 'Me, me, me; you, you, you' or 'Me, you; me, you.'

3 In screening the ball in football, try to keep your back towards the attacker with ball remote from attacker's side.

Group Practices and Small-sided Games

Team passing

In team passing, the goal is to make sets of 4 passes, without loss. Good dodging is essential to find a good space in which to receive the ball. Faking, as if to pass one way then passing a different way, should be tried here. Defenders should mark a player each and be a 'big' nuisance by spreading arms and legs wide to prevent passing or receiving.

Free-netball

In free-netball, good spacing can be imposed by limiting some players' movements, for example to own half of court, or defenders must be passive, allowing passes to be made without interference in own half of the court.

Floor-football

Flattish ball helps the floor-football by rolling away less often.

Lesson Plan 6 • 30-45 minutes
February

Warm-up and Footwork Practices
4–6 minutes

1 In your running, emphasise 'straight ahead' action of head, legs, arms and shoulders.

2 Tag, where the 6 starting chasers in coloured bands can catch you if you are running about within the lines. You can take refuge and be safe on a line. When caught take a coloured band and become a chaser. Be good sports and don't hide for too long on a line.

Skills Practices: with hockey sticks and balls
8–12 minutes

Partner practices

1 Push-pass, 5 or 6 metres apart, and move to a new position to receive your next pass.
   Emphasise:
   a feet sideways to direction of push and shoulder width apart
   b ball between feet and level with front foot
   c stick placed behind ball and pushed, no sound of stick on ball
   d stick kept low at end of stroke.

2 Side by side, dribble slowly forwards. On signal 'Push!' stop dribbling, push gently ahead of partner (illustrated) who now continues dribbling slowly and carefully, waiting for signal to 'Push!'

Group Practices and Small-sided Games
15–22 minutes

Hockey tackling

One third of group do not have a ball. Those with a ball dribble in area trying to avoid tackles by those without a ball. Tell class about 'Obstruction rule': dribbler must not shield ball with body or turn to place body between ball and opponents. Keep feet facing the way you are going when tackler approaches.

Rugby-touch

4 or 5 a side. Score by placing ball down on opponents' line. When touched you must pass ball. You may pass forwards in own half, but only sideways or backwards in opponents' half. Run straight and fast until touched, to gain ground.

Change-bench-ball

4 or 5 a side, with chalk 'bench'. Goal is scored when you pass ball to team-mate on 'bench' then run to bench to change places with him. He must pass ball to team-mate on court before leaving bench. Challenge teams to agree rule to speed up play, for example only 1 pass is allowed in own half.

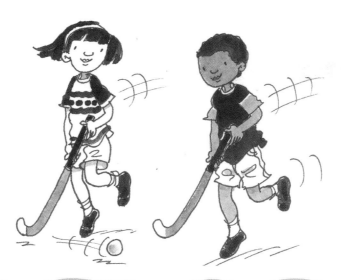

Games

Teaching notes and NC guidance
Development over 4–5 lessons

Lesson's main emphases:

a the NC general requirement to improve skills such as sending, receiving and travelling with a ball in invasion games.

b working individually in the warm-up, in pairs in the partner practices, in 4s (or 5s) in the games, to try to make this lesson almost non-stop. With the almost continuous action ensuring that no-one is cold, and with 3 varied games as the lesson's climax, it is hoped that there is something for everyone to look forward to, to enjoy while participating, and to reflect on with great pleasure.

Equipment: 30 hockey sticks and 15 small balls; 1 rugby ball; 1 large ball; chalk for marking the 'benches'.

Warm-up and Footwork Practices

1 Much running is spoiled by arms and shoulders twisting instead of pointing straight ahead. If you run along a line, your hands should remain parallel to the line, not cross it, as often happens.

2 If class stay on lines too long, becoming cold and not giving chasers a chance, the teacher should call 'All move!'

Skills Practices: with hockey sticks and balls

Partner practices

1 Emphasise that the push pass is literally a silent push with stick starting behind and touching ball. There must be no dangerous hitting with wild backswings of the stick.

2 In the change from dribbling to pushing the player has to move side on to the ball to make the push-pass to the partner.

Group Practices and Small-sided Games

Hockey tackling

In the introduction to tackling in hockey, one third of the class are allowed to try to 'steal' a ball by contacting the ball and trying to take it away. Those with the ball may not 'screen' it as you may do in football, but they can try to push ball past the would-be attacker and run around him.

Rugby-touch

In new-image rugby we must now pass the ball sideways or backwards in the opponents' half of the court. If the ball is passed forwards in the opponents' half, a 2-person scrum is formed. The ball is put into the scrum by a player of the non-infringing team, whose scrum teammate is the one who hooks it back into play.

Change-bench-ball

In cold weather particularly, change over the bench-catcher often. Encourage the catcher to be lively, on the move continuously, trying to position well for a variety of chest, overhead and bounce catches, moving from end to end of the 'bench'.

Lesson Plan 7 • 30–45 minutes
March

Warm-up and Footwork Practices
4–6 minutes

1 Running, using two thirds of netball court, slowly when near others, more quickly when space allows. Emphasise short rapid strides, forwards body lean and explosive arm action in sprinting.

2 Third of class in each third of court. Sprint to touch 4 sides of third, back to start. Run in a straight line, not in a circle. Repeat 2 or 3 times, with class final for regular winners in each group.

Skills Practices: with rugby balls or large balls
8–12 minutes

1 Triangle pass, 5 metres apart, 1 ball. A passes to B and runs to B's place as B passes to C and runs to C's place as C carries ball to what was A's place to re-start drill.

2 Lines of 3 running up and down court passing to each other along the line. Change middle person over often.

Invent a Game or Skills Practice
3–5 minutes

Invent a running, passing practice in 3s with 1 ball. (For example, lines of 3 run forwards. Middle person with ball passes to one side then runs behind that person who becomes new middle. He now passes and runs behind to other side.)

Group Practices and Small-sided Games
15–22 minutes

Rugby-touch

4 or 5 a side. Ball may be passed forwards in own half, but only sideways or backwards in opponents' half. Stress 'run fast and straight until touched' to gain ground. Team-mates must back up the player with the ball.

Playground-hockey

4 or 5 a side. Place ball on opponents' line to score. 2-touch hockey: receive on '1', find team-mate moving to space for pass on '2'. Defenders stay in own half for space. 1 rule to keep game moving, for example no dribbling in own half. Pass only.

Heading-ball

Large foam ball, 4 or 5 a side. After pass from team-mate, head ball over opponents' goal line to score. No running with ball. Pass and run forwards to advance ball for pass to a forehead when near opponents' line. A target person there can head or pass back.

Games

Teaching notes and NC guidance
Development over 4–5 lessons

Lesson's main emphases:

a the NC requirements to explore and understand the common skills and principles, including attack and defence, of invasion games, and to play fairly, compete honestly and demonstrate good sporting behaviour.

b remembering, as we come to the end of the winter Games programme, with its emphasis on lively running or invasion games, that teachers should be on the look out for, and be warm in their praise for, the many signs of achievement, improvement and success being enjoyed by so many children after about 6 months of working and practising hard. While these little games played in the small area of one third of a netball court might seem diminutive to the teacher, to the child who proudly says 'I have just scored my first ever try in rugby' the occasion is most important and memorable, and needs to be seen to be appreciated.

Equipment: 10 rugby or large balls; 10 hockey sticks and 1 ball; 1 large foam ball.

Warm-up and Footwork Practices

1 As primary school children become older we can ask them to work harder at more things for longer, and we keep the running going longer without stopping, plus asking them to be aware of spaces and to include short sprints in good style when space permits.

2 After the full warm-up and 2 or 3 sets of sprints we can ask them to reflect on how their bodies are feeling after the strong leg activity. 'Breathing deeply; feeling hot; whole body feels alive; slightly puffed out; feel wide awake, etc.'

Skills Practices: with rugby balls or large balls

'Sympathetic' is the expression often used of the way we pass to another to ensure a carefully aimed pass is sent at just the right speed and height for the runner to run on to. Turn your upper body right around towards the catcher.

Invent a Game or Skills Practice

Aim for continuous, whole court activity, with each group keeping very close, always aware of and never impeding other groups. Because we may run with the ball in this practice, it should be easy for Year 5 to refine it.

Group Practices and Small-sided Games

Rugby-touch

In new-image rugby, a 2-person scrum follows a pass forwards in the opponents' half. Non-offending team player puts ball at far foot of scrumming player in his team who is the only one allowed to hook it back.

Playground-hockey

In playground-hockey, encourage children to make up rules to help keep this difficult game moving without all encircling the ball 'like bees around a honey pot'. 'No tackling! One defender only may confront and the player must pass' is a good suggestion.

Heading-ball

Heading-ball attackers can try 'Plan 1 – get ball to head of target player for a header' or 'Plan 2 – get ball to target player who passes back to team-mate running in for a shot.'

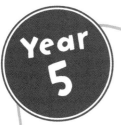

Year 5

Lesson Plan 8 • 30-45 minutes
April

Warm-up and Footwork Practices
4—6 minutes

1. Run and jump long or high, and continue running. In your long jump, swing your leading foot well forwards. In your upwards jump, swing your leading knee high up in front.

2. Free-and-caught. If caught by a chaser in coloured band, stand still, hands on head. Others can 'free' you by touching you on the elbow. Change chasers often.

Skills Practices: with large balls
8—12 minutes

Individual practices

Keep ball above head, throwing, catching, volleying. To volley, cup hands, palms clear of ball. Two thumbs and index fingers make a triangle through which you sight ball. Elbows slightly bent, knees bent. Strike and follow through on to toes.

Partner practices

2 metres apart only. Volley high and low to make partner move back, forwards and from side to side.

Invent a Game or Games Practice in 2s
3—5 minutes

Can you create a little game or practice to help you improve your volleying skills, sharing one ball? (For example, each in turn tries for a long rally, volleying ball straight up above head. Watching partner keeps count.)

Group Practices and Small-sided Games
15—22 minutes

Volleyball

1 ball between 2, rope 'net' between netball posts. Throw up to self and volley to partner. How long a rally can you make? No one-handers but you may volley up to 3 times on your side before sending it to your partner.

Long skipping ropes

Group skipping side to side, low or overhead, depending on ability and numbers (illustrated). Work out best way to learn long rope skipping. When do you enter rope?

4-player rounders

2 games. Children to decide on scoring, how out, number of balls bowled per batter.

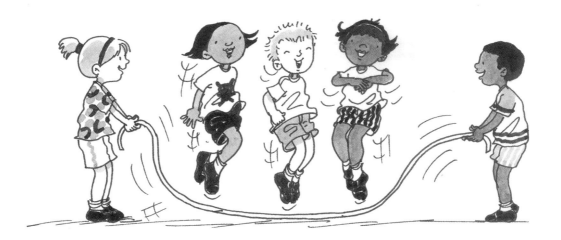

Games

Teacher notes and NC Guidance Development over 4–5 Lessons

Lesson's main emphases:

a the NC requirement to plan, perform and refine their own games and practices, working safely alone and with others.

b understanding that net and striking/fielding games are less active and vigorous than the invasion games. With young learners, these games can be static and inactive, and they should never be taught outdoors in cold winter weather. From April til July, during warmer weather, the emphasis is on teaching skills, small group practices and games of net and striking/fielding games. Since many of the NC requirements for athletic activities are also being pursued during summer months, it is essential that the children are trained to listen, respond, practise and work well and enthusiastically to cover as much work as possible. It is equally essential that schools totally reject the very common practice of 15-a-side rounders, often with the teacher bowling and 30 children spending an entire lesson learning nothing, practising nothing, hardly moving, and satisfying nothing within the NC. 15-a-side rounders, the commonly seen 'game' within summer term Physical Education, is the antithesis of all that good Physical Education stands for. It is neither physical nor educational and should be banned as a waste of precious time.

Equipment: 20 large balls; 3 long skipping ropes; 2 playbats and small balls and cones for rounders; long rope as 'net' for the volleyball.

Group Practices and Small-sided Games

Volleyball

Co-operative volleying practice over rope 'net' tied above head height of teacher. Emphasise the power that comes from the straightening of legs, elbows and the wrist-flick follow-through. Move early, receiving, to place body under ball in the settled down ready position with high arms ready. Aim ball above head of partner when you volley for an easy return.

Long skipping ropes

Groups of 4 or 5 with a long skipping rope. Come in when rope hits ground and is swinging away from you. Come out to left when rope swings to your right. With beginners, let the rope swing low from side to side only, not overhead.

4-player rounders

Limit area where ball may travel to that third of netball court. 6 turns for each batter, then all change around, seems a fair way to ensure that all experience all the activities.

Lesson Plan 9 • 30-45 minutes
May

Warm-up and Footwork Practices
4—6 minutes

1   Run and hurdle over lines in playground. Which is your leading leg in hurdling?

2   2s, sprint relay. Start back to back at centre of court with partner. On signal, one runs to nearer side line and back to touch partner who runs to line at his side. Who can touch 10 lines first?

Skills Practices: with small balls, bats and balls
8—12 minutes

Partner practices

Small balls

1   Aim at a line between you and count your good hits.

2   Stand close, throwing and catching underarm. Move a little further apart, and note the point when you start to throw overarm. Then start moving closer again.

Bat and ball

1   Balance ball on your bat; hit it up 3 times; then hit it to partner to see if he can catch it dead on bat; then repeat. Balance; strike up for 3; hit to partner.

2   8 metres apart, one strikes ball along ground for partner to run to field.

Invent a Game
3—5 minutes

Can you invent a game for 4 players with 1 bat and 1 ball, lines making a corner and a limited area? (For example, batter in corner strikes ball from own hand and calls name of the person who has to try to make a good catch. If successful, catcher takes bat.)

Group Practices and Small-sided Games
15—22 minutes

'Newcombe'

2 with 2, rope 'net' tied between netball posts. Throw ball over net to serve. Receiver catches in volley position before returning over net. How long a rally can your 4 make?

Non-stop cricket in 4s

2 games. Batter runs around skittle and back. Bowler may bowl at wicket even if batter not there. Change duties often.

Follow-the-leader

Choice of small or large balls, bat and ball, skipping rope, quoits or beanbags. Follow leader at about 2 metres and aim to develop a matching sequence in unison (illustrated). Can leader include 3 different actions?

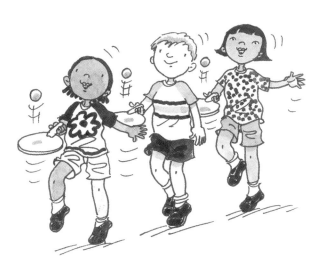

Teaching notes and NC guidance
Development over 4–5 lessons

Lesson's main emphases:

a the NC requirements to practise, adapt, improve and repeat longer and increasingly complex sequences of movement, and to improve the skills of sending and receiving a ball in striking/fielding games.

b putting the class in the picture, as always, about the contents of this lesson. 'The lesson this month includes athletic activity practices – running, hurdling, relays, throwing; striking/fielding games skills practices and game of non-stop cricket; net games practices in the game of Newcombe; and the opportunity to "develop your own games practices" with 1 bat and ball among 4 of you, and the follow-the-leader with a choice of equipment. The lesson is filled with variety and I hope that you all find something to enjoy very much. I also hope that you will all work hard, quietly and enthusiastically because we have a lot to do.'

Equipment: 15 bats and small balls; 5 large balls and long rope 'net' for Newcombe, cones or wickets for cricket, small and large balls, bats, ropes, beanbags, quoits for follow-the-leader.

Warm-up and Footwork Practices

1 In hurdling, leading leg goes up and down straight. Following leg trails to side, around and over imaginary hurdle. If it came straight through it would hit the hurdle.

2 For fair play's sake, all must run and touch the line before racing back to touch partner. Look out for and rebuke any who cheat by failing to touch the line, or who run off before the hand-touch from partner.

Skills Practices: with small balls, bats and balls

Partner practices

1 Small ball practices to develop aiming, throwing, catching, and the judgement of height, speed and distance vital in striking/fielding games.

2 In the bat and ball practices we are practising good timing and judgement of direction, force in sending a ball in striking/fielding games, and fielding a ball rolling towards you.

Invent a Game

The invented game or activity can be non-competitive, simply being practised to improve a difficult skill or, more likely, it will be competitive in a very limited court area, where the main consideration is to provide activity for all.

Group Practices and Small-sided Games

'Newcombe'

Newcombe is volleyball with the simplified skill of momentarily receiving the ball in the volley position before sending it.

Non-stop cricket in 4s

Bowl straight in non-stop cricket to force the batter to play and then run. This makes the game more lively with all active: fielding, backing up, waiting for return throw for run-out or to bowl again.

Follow-the-leader

In follow-the-leader, plan for a three-part, varied sequence. Can you repeat your little pattern together?

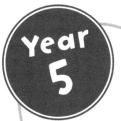

Lesson Plan 10 • 30-45 minutes
June

Warm-up and Footwork Practices
4–6 minutes

1   Run beside a partner, keeping together at same speed. Feel a good cruising rhythm that you can continue easily.

2   Now, by yourself, can you show me a three-step approach and a scissor jump over one of the many lines on the playground? 1, 2, 3 and swing up inside leg over the imaginary bar.

Skills Practices: with short-tennis rackets and balls and hoops
10–15 minutes

Individual practices

Short tennis
1   Walk with ball balanced on racket, strike it up, catch it dead.

2   Practise forehand and backhand strokes, side to side, over line.

Hoops
1   Can you spin the hoop on wrist, ankle or waist or on the ground to make it come back to you?

2   Try skipping with one or two hands on the hoop.

Partner practices

Short tennis
1   Partner throws for partner to hit back.

2   How long a rally of forehand hits can you make over a line 'net'?

Hoops
1   Can you bowl the hoop about 3 metres to your partner?

2   Can you and your partner make up a skipping routine together or alternately?

Group Practices and Small-sided Games
16–24 minutes

Short tennis

1 with 1. Working with, not against, your partner, how long a rally can you make? Serve by dropping ball and hitting it over net.

Tunnel-ball rounders

4 or 5 a side. Batting team all follow leader around diamond, scoring 1 point for every cone passed before fielders pass ball through legs to end of tunnel and shout 'Stop!' (illustrated)

Newcombe or quoits over rope 'net' tied between netball posts

Point is scored when ball or quoit lands on opponents' court or fails to clear net. Let children decide on a fair way to serve and when to change ends.

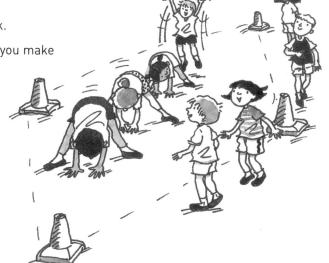

Games

Teaching notes and NC guidance
Development over 4–5 lessons

Lesson's main emphases:

a the NC requirements to develop an understanding of, and play small-sided versions of, recognised games, and to improve sending and receiving skills in net games.

b allocating a full 6 or 9 minutes at least to each of the 3 games of the final, most important part of the lesson for a satisfactory climax.

Equipment: 15 short-tennis rackets and balls; 15 hoops; long rope 'net' tied between netball posts for quoits or newcombe; 5 quoits or 5 large balls for net games.

Warm-up and Footwork Practices

1 In side-by-side running together, runner on the inside steps short on turns because outer partner's arc is greater. Try to 'feel' your steady cruising speed, running in unison.

2 Scissor jumping is slow and springy with the last, jumping stride a heel, ball, toes rocking up action. Bent leading knee and both arms swing up into the action.

Skills Practices: with short-tennis rackets and balls and hoops

Individual practices

Short tennis

1 To catch a ball 'dead', go up to meet it early, then let racket 'give' to catch ball without a rebound.

2 Shuffle side to side, playing gentle forehand and backhand shots up and over the line.

Hoops

1 Spin hoop on the spot. Now try throwing it away with back spin to make it come back.

2 Low swing from side to side with 1 hand is a good way to start skipping with a hoop before the difficult overhead swings.

Partner practices

Short tennis

1 Encourage a side on to partner position when striking, so racket easily faces intended direction of hit. From ready position facing partner, turn to one side or other. Take racket well back, ready to hit ball at top of bounce when opposite you.

2 Rally gently at about 5 metres from the line, trying to hit ball to about 2 metres in front of partner.

Hoops

1 Hold top of hoop steady with non-bowling hand. Bowl it by pulling with a flat hand on top of hoop.

2 The skipping routine can include skipping with hoop flat on ground.

Group Practices and Small-sided Games

Short tennis

In co-operative short tennis, aim to land ball just short of partner's forehand to make the return easy, leading to long rallies. Take racket back early and turn for a 'side on' hit.

Tunnel-ball rounders

In tunnel-ball rounders, the ball is struck by hand forwards and must remain within the third of the netball court. Fielding player who receives ball stands and lets team-mates form a tunnel behind him. Last one in tunnel calls 'Stop!'

Newcombe or quoits over rope 'net' tied between netball posts

Competitive quoits or Newcombe, where 5-point games are played before changing ends. Much decision-making by children about rules and scoring systems should be encouraged.